INHERITANCE

by Kelley M. Moore

PREFACE

This is a mother's story.

The story is extraordinary. Or is it?

The story comes from a million different memories documented from a lifetime of dancing around the truth and waiting for the next shoe to drop.

You may have just thought of a similar experience that you might have had along your way, dancing that same dance, and waiting for that same shoe.

We are different, but we can learn. Anything is possible. We do recover.

This is my journey.

Chapter 1

The Pediatrician
Saturday February 19, 2005

Our two daughters were in high school and, as far as we believed, they were very busy in their school life. Our oldest was involved in field hockey and friends. Our youngest was inseparably immersed in the drama club. I was working, running a family business, and held a second full-time position as a program director for a local non-profit organization. My husband had taken employment as the president of a local non-profit business organization as well, in addition to being the payroll administrator and chief bottle washer for our business. We were working hard, hopeful that both daughters would attend college one day. I always wanted that for my girls.

With adolescents comes a bit of chaos, some arguing, a few secrets, a fib here and there, possibly some white blatant lies, and, of course, a couple of groundings for broken curfews. Right?

The atmosphere in our home was a bit darker.

There was an uninvited presence in our home. It had been there for a very long time. I cannot remember when it moved in. The timing of its arrival had been glossed over.

After years of living on the edge and waiting day after day for the next shoe to drop, something was bubbling to the surface, like the potato water in the pot on top of the stove. That starchy, thickened liquid that's scalding hot and boils over, searing the burner with a relentless hissing. You cannot get to the stove fast enough to stop it. Living on the edge is like the tiny shards of broken glass that pierce your skin at every swipe to rid them. You can't feel the slicing swords, but you're bleeding.

My husband and I, along with our girls, knew there was a monster living among us that had been holding us captive. Of course, we knew it. The screaming of its unforsaken silence was like a criminal predator.

We could feel it.

All the cynical attention was pointing to our youngest.

As parents, we had done our research. We thought we had kept a tight grip. We had made the right connections with the local police department. We viewed all the calls on her cell phone. We made psychiatrist appointments for the whole family. My daily trips to the high school were enough to spread unease throughout the school staff, as well as to some parents who, like me, wanted to believe that their child was nothing but stellar.

In 2003, one of the teachers at the high school accused me of child neglect and child abuse. My husband and I were subjected to a review and home visit from the State Department of Children Services. Following the merciless digging through layers of questioning within the family interviews, the claim was withdrawn by the case manager. During the visit his report was finalized:

CHILD	ALLEGATION	PERPETRATOR	CONFIRMATION STATUS
Daughter	Physical Abuse	Mother	Not Substantiated
Daughter	Physical Neglect	Mother	Not Substantiated

"Your case will be closed at this time."

As scary as the state's home visit experience was, nothing was more invasive or intrusive than when my youngest and I had arrived at the appointment I had scheduled with the family pediatrician. Yes, you read that right, pediatrician.

The doctor knew something was not quite right as well.

The doctor instructed my daughter to go into the office bathroom and urinate in a cup for a drug test. As cool as a cucumber and as silent as a lamb, she strutted her way to the bathroom. Shortly after she exited the bathroom with confidence, she handed the full cup of bodily waste to the medical assistant.

I was shaking.

She sat stoically.

As we waited for the doctor to return to the room we were in, all I could hear was the deafening pound coming from the wall clock each time the secondhand passed by every moment within that sixty-minute cycle.

Every moment.

We waited.

And waited.

After what felt like years, though I am sure was only minutes, the good doctor came back into the examining room. She stood directly in front of my youngest daughter, staring down at her without a blink while she spoke to me. In the most unapologetic fashion, and very sure of herself, the doctor announced that it was clear to her that my daughter needed to be watched while she "peed." Apparently, she could not be trusted in the bathroom alone. The doctor reported that the urine sample had been diluted with water, presenting an inaccurate outcome. I was then instructed to follow my seventeen-year-old daughter, the pediatrician's patient, into the bathroom and literally witness her fill a second urine sample cup as she sat on the toilet. I followed right behind her to the closet-like restroom. I obeyed my orders with a heavy heart and a knot in my stomach.

I was still shaking.

As the yellow trickle of bodily waste consumed the second plastic cup, no words were exchanged between my daughter and myself. As she peed and I watched, she still appeared as stoic as before.

Or was it ice cold?

Finally, we both emerged from the tiny bathroom. My daughter was holding the warm sample, and again passed the container to the medical assistant. Back in the examination room we went to wait for a second toxicology result, which would presumably be more accurate than the watered-down sample.

Caught.

In. Plain. Sight.

I could not breathe.

That damn clock.

I remember the pediatrician returning to the sterile room that we continued to occupy. She delivered the true result of the final sample of excrement that I was forced to watch flow into the cup. The test had undeniably produced an obscene amount of cocaine levels in the urine sample. Without hesitation, the pediatrician recommended that we contact a local treatment center for an assessment. From there we would receive suggestions with next steps for adolescent drug abuse treatment immediately.

I needed my inhaler.

I contacted my husband as we made our way to the elevator from the third floor of the medical building. I told him that he needed to meet us at home. He left his office immediately. She and I drove home in complete silence. Both of us sat staring directly outward through the windshield for the twenty-five-minute drive.

I felt as though I had been hit by a truck.

When my husband got home, we sat in the living room together, watching our baby girl stare at the floor. The long battle that had grown so fierce and more threatening day to day, month to month, from year to year, had finally brought my baby to a complete breakdown. She cried that she could no longer live her double life. She pleaded for forgiveness and understanding. She admitted to being in a place that she didn't know how to get out of.

She was giving up.

It was at that moment I had lost all sense of time.

I remember running out of the room to throw up. Suddenly, I realized why I felt like I was living with my brother, as though it hadn't been in my face every single day.

In a way, I was.

Surrendered.

Out loud.

In. Plain. Sight.

Yet there we were.

Chapter 2

Intake

The next day, the assessment was completed at the local center. The result brought us to a place that we were drowning in. We were referred to an out-of-state program for drug and alcohol treatment for adolescents, where children stay until they are well enough to be discharged back home. The therapist told us that a "bed" would be available in five days.

"A bed will be available…" What did any of that even mean?

There was a constant buzz in my head that would make me dizzy and gasping for air.

Where were we as a family? The thought of one of my babies living so far away from home when she needed me most was difficult for me to comprehend. How was it that a mother could not help her youngest daughter?

How?

The only thing I could do was fall in line like a good soldier and march forward with what the professionals were telling us. While we waited for that precarious call, I slept with her on the floor of my bedroom every night of those days. On the morning of day five, the phone rang. That "bed was available."

I felt queasy.

We got in the car, as ordered, and drove two and a half hours to another abyss.

We arrived at our destination. I could not get out of the car right away. I sat in the passenger seat, staring through the windshield again. I couldn't figure out if the outside of the building was inviting or not.

Just staring.

Our baby was the first one out of the car. Then my husband. I had to take a deep breath to find the door handle and push myself out from under the seat belt. The hours that we traveled drove me into one of the most self-isolated, frightening, and truthful moments in my life.

At that time, I was a forty-five-year-old mother of two girls. Our oldest daughter was a freshman in college, living in a dormitory with roommates. Here we were in a place so far away from home with my youngest daughter. She was in the final months of her senior year of high school. We weren't even sure if graduating was in the cards for her or not. She didn't know, either.

I was holding literature that was given to us at the assessment center. The cover of the flyer read, "Treatment Programs for Chemical Dependency—Inpatient and Outpatient Services for Adolescents and Adults." It could have been in an entirely different language because I was suffocating anyway.

I had never even heard of this kind of place.

Treatment Programs? This was a place for other people.

Yet there we were.

We pushed through the one-million-pound door. We were greeted by someone. I suppose she might have been nice. I couldn't hear her, anyway.

The walls were yellow from old cigarette smoke. The glass-enclosed office area felt like a violation of my privacy. We were exposed to everyone there as they attempted to take a glimpse of the "new admit." The cruddy-colored metal desks were cluttered with other people's history and other people's information. I felt as though I was imposing on other family's vulnerable moments that were captured in time. I remember feeling helpless and detached from reality.

Yet there we were.

Our turn.

On March 2, 2005, my husband turned forty-nine years old. Our youngest daughter was being processed through the Intake procedure for residential treatment for drug and alcohol abuse.

Intake.

Intake would be a term that I would become all too familiar with.

I remember shivering, yet it was seventy degrees.

My husband, one of the strongest men and best fathers I knew, sat at one of those cold metal desks. The distance between him and I seemed like a football field. He was filling out our personal, medical, and confidentiality forms; all to be included on top of the unkempt array of other people's stories. His strained gaze looked toward me as I was fixed on him.

Watching him.

He was in shock.

I wanted to support him. My lips formed the words "Happy Birthday." He just stared back at me with a blank look. I wondered if he could even see me. Was he looking at me? Was he in there? What was he staring at?

I stared back.

We were overcome with a weight that felt so debilitating. The silence was deafening.

Staring.

Waiting. Waiting. Waiting.

My eyes found the nerve to slowly scan the two-by-four unkempt cell that the three of us had been confined to.

There she was.

Our baby.

Just like that.

Right before our very eyes and in plain sight.

As though there were no signs, nothing to notice, no hints or ideas, no thoughts, or not any inclination that "something" was off. Chaos had become such a dysfunctional part of our family routine that the awareness of when it had all begun, the date of arrival of the forever tug of an ugly war, was blurred, glossed over.

My baby looked so small. She was so tiny sitting against that dirty wall. She looked lost, defeated but humble. Tired and surrendered. Her body appeared so weak. She melted into the chipped plaster as though she might be able to go unnoticed. Like in a vacuum, I remember being sucked back into a memory when she turned five years old.

~~~~~~~~~~~~~~~~

There were six family members that had gotten together for a birthday ride on a dinner train for our little girl that was turning five years old. Dinner was in the moving dining car and we all sat in anticipation of the Happy Birthday song that would accompany the birthday cake.
~~~~~~~~~~~~~~~~

None of us could wait to see the look on that baby face when she realized that the big surprise cake was for her.

The wait staff gathered and proceeded down to our table. They began to sing the traditional song everyone loves on anyone's special day. The train staff, so delightfully, encouraged the rest of the dinner guests to sing along to the little birthday girl. She was sitting so politely in the best of the best birthday dresses. Her legs were crossed on top of the leather seat, so she could see above the table. Her hands were folded like a princess on top of the table.

Suddenly, my memory became so clear.

How had I not seen it then?

My five-year-old quickly shot me a look. I smiled back at her with a comforting grin and sang in chorus with everyone else. I was trying to soothe the look of fear and discomfort all over her face that I thought I had just identified. I reached out to her with a facial expression of safety.

Without notice, and with an innocent declaration of surrender, she put her head down, ever so slowly, right on those adorable ten little fingers that were folded on top of that table.

The song was over. The entire train car was applauding as the five pink candles flickered. The audience patiently waited for the birthday girl to blow out her candles as she held the coveted center of attention. Eventually, all the other dinner guests giggled a bit and returned to their own private celebrations.

She never lifted her head.

I put my hand on the top of her hair and softly moved my hand down to her tiny, tiny shoulder. I whispered in her ear that it was okay to sit up and blow out her candles.

There was no response. Her head down.

Nothing.

I nudged her a bit to grasp her attention. I thought that maybe she hadn't heard me offer her the rite of passage to own the privilege bestowed to a birthday girl who could wish for anything in her whole world.

Again, no response. Head down.

Again, nothing.

I softly placed my cheek to hers to have a private conversation with her when I realized that she was sleeping. Out cold. Just like that.

I was stunned and taken aback but brushed the episode aside.

Eventually, I was able to wake her with encouraging prompts. I offered her the piece of cake that held one last burning candle with its pink and white colors sliding slowly down the waxy spiral.

She responded.

"No thank you."

Twelve years later, my eyes were fixed on that seventeen-year-old broken sweetheart across that dank, dark space of an office I felt hostage to. In that moment, I silently questioned that dinner train event back on her fifth birthday. Had my baby girl literally and completely checked out of her own self-pressured reality?

She never had another piece of cake.

~~~~~~~~~~~~~~~~

The clinical staff person, at this place meant for others, explained to us that the plan was that our daughter was going to be admitted for a twenty-eight-day treatment program for alcohol and cocaine addiction. We were informed that her progress would be measured daily. We were told that her minimum stay would be for two weeks but that ongoing evaluations would determine her complete treatment stay.

What did any of it mean?

I was feeling so disconnected from myself. I recall that I could hear people speaking. I remember seeing their mouths moving, however I had no idea what anyone was saying.

Little did we know how much we would learn about the power of the insurance companies and the unequivocal faith we offer to such companies when we really feel like prisoners. Insurance companies were always so confusing, anyway, and now we had to depend on several strangers who were telephonic caseworkers that would read from a
~~~~~~~~~~~~~~~~

piece of paper from a million miles away. He or she reported the information to another caseworker, a dozen more million miles away, as though any one of them knew anything about my baby.

As though any of them knew anything about us.

Strangers.

Haunting.

Yet there we were.

INHERITANCE

Chapter 3

Admission

Following the numerous dialogue and paperwork that seemed endless, our daughter was about to be led away by the treatment center employees who were complete strangers to us.

The three of us embraced each other with fierce gravity and tears in our eyes. We were overwhelmed and exhausted. I felt as though she and I were seeing each other for the first time. As though there were no hints or no clues of any kind she had been continuously crying out for help. It was then that it had occurred to me, that I probably had not seen her eyes looking straight at me in years. We were lost and fearful. We felt empty. We felt unfastened from our own reality with utter disbelief.

We were broken.

She was broken.

Surreal.

I was numb.

I couldn't feel my face.

My eyes were swollen.

Funny, what life throws at you. We thought we knew everything we needed to know about our baby. Apparently, we did not, and we lived with her in the same house. In plain sight. Strangers would get to know more about her than we did.

What had I been doing all those years? Where was I? Where was she?

In my mind, I couldn't help but see the five-year-old little birthday girl on that dinner train. I couldn't unsee that five-year-old's plea for something from across the dinner table that day. I clearly had misunderstood. What I saw as a mere surprise just might have been a silent shout out for help because of becoming the unexpected center of attention.

How had she really felt that day on that train? On her fifth birthday?

Yet there we were.

We left our baby with strangers. We had always said, and "Stranger Danger" was always taught, "Do not go with strangers." We had just traveled over two and half hours to leave her with strangers. I could not get that fact out of my head and heart. The journey felt so right when we had backed out of the driveway from home but at that moment, a million miles away, it felt so wrong.

I remember questioning myself over and over. What was I doing to my baby? Did I know anything about this place that we were told to bring her to "for her own good"? Did that place, meant for others, include my daughter?

It all felt so opposite, so backwards.

Backwards.

I couldn't say for exactly how long we held on to each other, but it felt like a lifetime. In a strange sort of way, it felt like a farewell to an old friend that we knew we would never see again. Without realizing it, perhaps it was.

We had to let go.

The man took her. The door slammed shut. We were severed from our baby and the new world that she would embrace.

My husband and I just stood there, staring at that dungeon of a door that exploded shut like a metal boom diminishing anything that could have or would have been of any comfort.

She was on one side of that door with strangers. We were on the other.

I'd be lying if I said that I knew how long we stood there staring at that dirty, scratched rock-solid violating blockade. I don't.

Our youngest was gone. Just like that.

At some point, we had to realize that there were ugly bold, black letters on that ugly dark gateway into God knows where staring back at us. We couldn't quite comprehend what the capitalized letters were that seemed to be shouting at us from that institutional barricade.
Then we focused.

"PATIENTS ONLY BEYOND THIS POINT."

We gripped each other's hands tightly enough to tingle as though hanging on for dear life. We did find a thirst for air and never looked at each other. We turned and exited the building.

Silent.

We would later learn that our seventeen-year-old daughter, following the admission process, my baby was offered a legal document that her underage signature would allow the treatment center staff to hold all information about her treatment from us, her parents. We would have no right to updates or any progress that she was making to be able to return home. What that meant was that following her authorization with her underage signature, the treatment center would no longer "Confirm or Deny" that she was even a patient there.

Privacy policies, HIPPA Regulations.

Betrayal.

I would begin a relationship with silence that I had never considered before. I was learning to listen differently, something I thought I had done so well.

Chapter 4

Addiction Chooses
Someone
Anyone
Everyone

Suppose the title of the chapter read something like any one of the following:

"Cancer Chooses," or "Heart Failure Chooses," or "Kidney Failure Chooses."

Chances are there would be a sense of warmth or a touch of empathy that may come over the reader. Maybe there would be a feeling of sorrow as to an unexpected path that a patient and a patient's family will endure.

A diagnosis from a doctor.

Someone you may know. Perhaps someone you are related to. Yourself.

Your child.

Not one person ever chooses the disease of cancer. Nor does anyone choose heart disease or that of kidney disease. Can it be possible that each disease chooses that one person, and maybe for a variety of reasons? It may be an undiagnosed symptom or a particularly challenging time in one's life, or just maybe one's pure bad luck. Most times no one understands why.

Maybe, it's hereditary.

Would anyone believe that just like any other disease that shows up uninvited, totally unexpected, and one that can possibly kill you, may also include the disease of addiction?

Addiction chooses someone.

Anyone. And then everyone.

Just like that.

Right before our very eyes and in plain sight, we unrealistically believe that cocaine, alcohol, diet pills, heroin, Adderall, oxycontin, Xanax, ecstasy, marijuana, fentanyl (I can go on) just show up.

Just like that.

As though there were no signs, nothing to notice, no hints or ideas, no thoughts, or not one inclination that "something" is off.

Chaos becomes an unnatural part of the family routine and, somehow, the awareness, the date of arrival of the forever tug of an ugly war, goes unseen and undetected. The timing of the hostile invasion is completely glossed over.

But is it?

There are questions and demands that we take to bed every single night following the crescendo of combative, terribly confusing, and suffocating episodes. The questions are forcibly thrown from you like darts to a bullseye.

"How could you do this to us?"
"Who do you think you are?"
"Look how much we have done for you."
"I didn't bring you up to behave like this! Why are you lying?"

Just to name a few.

I remember the question that invaded my head over and over and over again most nights during those unsettling years in my own home, with my own youngest daughter.

"Why do I feel like I am living with my brother?"

It was like a broken record or that annoying sound of someone's fingernails slowly descending the entire length of a chalk board.

Does anyone pay attention?

Neither a daughter, a son, your sister, a brother, a dad, a mom, an aunt, an uncle, a cousin, a best friend, a grandfather, nor a grandmother ever woke up saying to themselves, "Yup. Self-destruction is on my 'to-do' list today. Today is the day I am going to ruin my entire life, all my healthy relationships, and every bit of trust from all the people I love. That's it. I want to ruin my reputation, my character, everything I know to be right, kind, and just. I'm going to throw that all away. Today."

No one ever says that.

My daughter never said that, either.

Nor did my brother or my father. My two grandfathers didn't, either.

Just like any other disease.

Addiction Chooses.

Someone.

Anyone.

Everyone.

Chapter 5

In. Plain. Sight.

When I look back at those years prior to the weakening surrender, the truth was that my daughter's relationship with drugs and alcohol was not as silent as her world and her mind had convinced her. The dirty little secret was as loud as ever to everyone in her limited view of verity. Everyone she encountered knew exactly what she was doing to herself and what was happening to her. Friends would report horrific stories to their parents. The parents would then whisper amongst themselves and tell their children to keep away. Teachers would have conversations in the staff room while drinking their morning coffee, discussing the perceived notion that my daughter was getting abused and neglected at home, which was a perception as to why she was so thin. The secret that she thought she was keeping so well, exposed itself as an intruder that took up every ounce of attention from everyone.

In. Plain. Sight.

An unwanted behavior and toxic, invisible boarder eased into our lives silently and undetected at first. Then, somewhere along the line and without any formal introduction, the dark havoc we were living as a family couldn't be ignored. I couldn't determine when the innocence of adolescence ceased and the tangled web of tension, lies, and deceit began. It was apparent that life, as we had come to accept as volatile and disruptive, had changed all of us into mistrusting, secretive, and sad beings. We couldn't see each other but lived in the same house.

The gray area.

Could it get any worse?

Life as we knew it...Which life?

Long ago were the days of the youngest little girl pulling on my neck to be sure to place her cheek to mine so we could feel each other's smiles. I would inhale the wonderful, soft, clean, baby powder smell that only a mother could detect. The only life I had come to know was nothing short of combative, skeptical, sick, punitive, sad, and exhausting, yet, still, she was a baby.

My baby.

The older sister, away at college, would be able to be spared this turmoil, or so I thought. Little did I know that the coming change was for all of us. The change that would be bestowed on us would replace the chaotic existence we had become so accustomed to have lived by. We had all forgotten what it was like to appreciate one another, listen to one another, and most importantly, love one another.

The fear for all of us was the unknown. What we did understand was that something had shifted, and it wasn't going to be easy.

Nothing was easy.

The shift would change me.

The shift would change all of us.

Chapter 6

July 26, 1987, 2:15 a.m.

Life was the way it was supposed to be, right? Fourteen hours of labor with our oldest daughter—normal. After dancing in the delivery room for a second time, while in a welcomed and expected contraction discomfort, we were ready to take on another newborn that would bring our family to a total of four, just as we had planned. Five hours of labor would be the extent of our second daughter's introduction to the world.

July 26, 1987, at 2:15 a.m., was the miraculous moment that the sister sibling arrived.

But something was off.

She didn't cry.

You know, the sound that every mom, dad, doctor, nurse, and everyone else in the delivery room waits for at the final push into life.

That. Didn't. Happen.

She didn't cry.

I remember sitting up from that God-awful delivery table with a horrific panic in my voice.

"She isn't crying, why isn't she crying?"

I stared at my husband, my rock, and begged why. I wanted to know what was happening. He didn't know, either. Our baby was so swiftly swept away from us by the tending nurses. The only thing left behind them was an obvious silence. My doctor hurried into the room and tried to offer us words that seemed reasonable and scientific. What did we know about anything other than the first breath of life that was absent in the room. We hadn't even had a name for her yet. My baby would never experience the gift that comes within the first seconds of life. The first warm touch that comes from the mother. I was deprived of the gift that solidifies the first connection between mother and child.

What did any of this mean?

We would find out exactly what the dreaded silence meant.

Doctors would meet with us soon after the birth to explain that our new baby was born with a type of heart disorder, and that heart specialists were being called in from one of the biggest children's hospitals in the state. The diagnosis would later determine that the baby's heart rate would slow down at some point, and then begin to race, resulting in the heart skipping a beat, trying to catch up with itself and return to a normal pace.

There was so much that we didn't know or understand. There was an overload of emotion and questions about what the future would hold. I remember my husband walking the hospital halls with an empty plastic water pitcher in his hand on the off chance that he would need to use it to expel every ounce of anxiety and fear that had built up in such a short amount of time. The dancing we had done in the delivery room suddenly felt so far away.

I finally got to hold my baby following her jump into life, as delayed as it was. We all did. Her older sister included. That nineteen-month old sister kept that little sibling under her baby wing, as though we had brought something home from the hospital just for her. The baby sister was claimed as her own.

After a month of monitoring closely, the heart disorder had diminished and was back to normal. Life would resume, as it was supposed to, right?

Heart Disorder Chose my baby.

A daughter's Christmas gift from Elementary School.

Dear Mom.

As a Christmas present I would like to tell you how much I'm thankful for you.

As I asked myself what I'm thankful for, was it a toy, was it food or was it family? Yes it was it was my mom! I'm going to tell you how close you are to me, how you've always been there for me in many way's, and how we've always been truthful to eachother.

My mom and I are very close. We've always felt comfortable together. Because are friendship is very stronge. I've always felt close to her the most. Even when I got punished I would try to relieve what I did wrong, because I believed that most of the time I was the one who was wrong! She was and still is a very important person in my life!

My mom has always been there for me no matter what. When I would play a game or a sport and lose she would always come in with a positive mind to cheer me up. When I was little, I would have bad dreams and end up running into her room, she would try to explain how your mind still works while your sleeping. Then she would let me sleep next to her and my dad, Or she would try to put me asleep by talking to me in my bed. She's been supportive and there for me.

My mom and I have also been very truth-ful. I could always tell her anything. I know there are no secrets between us. I think that's a very special thing to have. And I'm lucky to have that relationship. To have that feeling, actually knowing that anything can be told is comf-forting.

I am very close to my mom. She's always been there for me and we're very truthful. I hope someone in your life reflection on your life because it's very comforting. It's a very lucky thing to have.

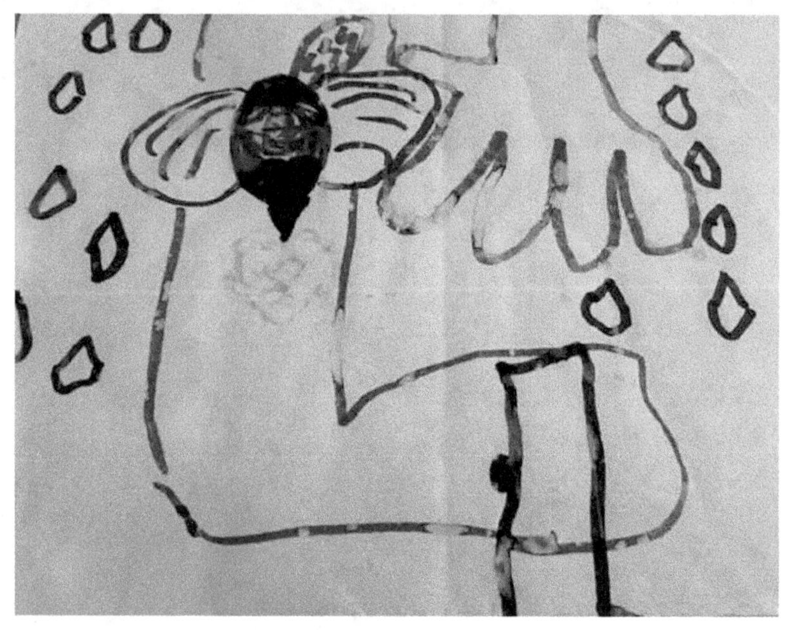

Chapter 7

It's. Gray.

The "gray area" is defined as ***"an area or situation in which it is difficult to judge what is right and what is wrong."***

The gray area feels backwards, opposite.

When the disease of addiction snuck into our lives undetected, what day was that?

There's a belief that the dirty, unfathomable behavior came without notice. The signs are ignored and sometimes justified or redefined. Looking back, would anyone believe that, sometimes, the disease of addiction gets swept under someone's ripped-up rug, only denying the reality that everyone is being affected?

Denial.

Just like cancer or heart disease, even kidney disease.

Just like a heart disorder.

How is it that the cry for help is missed or, better yet, misunderstood?

The Disease of Addiction Chooses. Someone.

Anyone. Everyone.

Then we all fall victim to a character, a part in the play that no one ever auditioned for. We refuse to see the nasty truth for what it is, in plain sight, but we all take a role like a pro.

I learned about all the roles performed by families affected by the disease of addiction. Through a multitude of books and literature I couldn't get enough of and weekly appointments with my very own psychiatrist, family group therapy sessions I was thirsty for, I was enlightened to the fact that the disease of addiction chooses everyone in its path. Everyone plays a role.

Everyone.

There is a Star in the family.

He or she is the more responsible and could also be called the hero. The Star is most often another teenager in the house who may also be the oldest. The Star is probably an overachiever who represents themselves as happy and carefree when what the Star is doing is hiding their own sadness.

~~~~~~~~~~~~~~

True to form, that was our oldest daughter. She never had to study for an exam. She always performed in theater. She loved joining the supreme high school choral groups and excelled in sports as well. However, she also lived the constant whispers throughout the high school hallways while a junior and her younger sister, a freshman. She was exposed to the lies and rumors that were spreading, making it difficult for the two sisters to look each other in the face as they crossed each other's paths. As the oldest sibling, she also felt helpless to understand any of what was happening involving her sister. The only way she could respond was with anger and distrust.

Like my older sister, second born, the middle child, the protector, the smart one.

It's a gray area.

~~~~~~~~~~~~~~

The Lost Child is another role.

The Lost Child looks everywhere to fit in, whether or not the Lost Child is aware of that decision they have made for themselves. The Lost Child stays silent, so as not to add one more chaotic existence to the already futile environment that controls everyone in the house.

~~~~~~~~~~~~~~
~~~~~~~~~~~~~~

I don't know if my husband was ever lost, as such, but he took on the quiet role. A businessman by profession, a great father and husband, he was always observing, listening, strategizing, and always trying to understand what was at hand. Someone once referred to him as "Being silently everywhere." That description was pretty accurate at work and at home.

~~~~~~~~~~~~~~~~

The Enabler, more times than none, exists within the family affected by the disease of addiction.

The Enabler is the person who makes excuses for the active addict, finding some level of justification for the dysfunction within the family. Sometimes the Enabler parent or spouse finds themselves paying for the consequences of the individual struggling from the disease of addiction. While covering up all the imperfections of the loved one who struggles, the Enabler adds to the growing sickness by clouding anger with the act of financial assistance. The Enabler believes that their actions are helping, when in fact the message to the one who struggles with the disease of addiction is that they will be taken care of no matter how bad it gets. Active addiction remains.

Such a scenario might look something like this: A parent or spouse who allows their loved one who is struggling to live in the home rent free. The Enabler may be paying all the bills for the adult or child. That same, well-intended being might be driving the person who is struggling with the Disease of Addiction to unknown destinations in a part of town that otherwise they would not find themselves in. Lest we not forget that the Enabler might just be causing a more debilitating outcome for that sick
~~~~~~~~~~~~~~~~

individual. The person struggling from the Disease of Addiction then learns nothing, has no real-life consequences to the real-life mishaps that adult living sometimes endures. Whether it's alcohol, cocaine, marijuana, or heroin, you know the list, somehow, the Enabler may be allowing the substance to win over what we all know to be right.

It's a gray area.

~~~~~~~~~~~~~~~~

Then there is the Comedian.

The Comedian offers a diversion from the hostile environment with a type of comic relief. Everything is funny. There is a joke for just about anything most of the time. When the attention is being drawn to the Comedian in the family, nothing must be wrong with the whole. When in actuality, hurt and broken have consumed the entire family unit, yet covering that up somehow feels awkwardly right.

Gray.

There was no laughter going on in our home, but clearly that had been my role while I was growing up and, still, when my nephews were young, too.

~~~~~~~~~~~~~~~~

I believe that when our oldest went to college, she must have thought that she was finally safe and away from all the pandemonium and mayhem.

Was she, though?

I look back and I am reminded of her four-year college career that had somehow morphed into a five-year stint. I remember her father and me taking a trip to her college dorm to investigate the reason behind grades being so poor and why classes were being missed. Sadly, today, as I write this memoir, it occurs to me that the behavior was possibly known as the role of Scapegoat. The Scapegoat suffers by falling into "if you can't beat 'em, join 'em."

She wasn't safely away from the havoc that became the routine amongst the tender years of growing up. Havoc followed her.

Still gray.

Any role that takes the attention away from the obvious heartache and fear will work for the masquerade that plays out. The ever-so-obvious struggle, the "how to cope" frustrations along with the "how do I get back to real life?" plan never get brought to the light soon enough. The mere dysfunction that the Disease of Addiction inflicts on the entire family, keeping everyone captive to the darkness, goes unspoken, only to dig everything and everyone deeper into a black hole.

The Disease of Addiction Chooses. Someone.

Anyone. Everyone.

<div align="center">~~~~~~~~~~~~~~</div>

March 2, 2005

Your sister and I bought these bracelets for each of us on Saturday. We wanted you to have this one so that all three bracelets can be a symbol of a new beginning. Every time we look at these on our wrists, we will be reminded of all our commitments toward positive mental and physical health. They are magnetic, which symbolizes how all of us, including Dad, are drawn to support one another. It won't be easy, but we can do this together. We look forward to your safe return home. We love you very much. Please remember that.

Mom, Dad and your sister.

~~~~~~~~~~~~~~~~
~~~~~~~~~~~~~~~~

Chapter 8

Family Therapy Day, March 3, 2005
Part 1

It was Thursday March 3, 2005. We had made the two-and-a-half hour drive home the night before. We were drained.

At about 8:15 a.m., we received a phone call from an out-of-state phone number. Another stranger. The stranger said that she was the Director of Family Services for the treatment center we had just left our baby with. She explained that parents and loved ones of patients were expected to participate in the Family Therapy Day, which was offered once a month. She informed us that the monthly group session was scheduled for 10:00 a.m. that morning and advised us to get on the road as soon as possible, being that the distance from our home to the treatment center was an almost three-hour drive.

We were so aware of the miles separating us.

We left immediately.

We arrived back at the treatment center within moments of the beginning of the session. Another stranger, who identified himself as one of the adolescent counselors, reported that my baby would be arriving with the other patients soon.

In twenty-four hours, we had traveled back and forth and back again to this place meant for other people and, somehow, it felt like it had been decades since we had left her there. We couldn't wait to see her.

I was afraid.

We were informed that there was a total of seventy families as well as friends of "addicts" that would be participating in the session.

Addicts.

Next, like cattle being guided by a farmer and his tractor, we were ushered towards a staircase that descended downward. I witnessed each family clinging onto each other at each turn of the stairwell; no one knowing what to expect.

I held onto my rock.

We were all escorted into this massive room with the same yellow walls as the ones we had been surrounded by just the day before. We stood

on a thin, discolored carpet that was torn in some places. The mangy rug spread out under our feet from wall to wall, offering no comfort. On the ceiling were rows and rows of sterile fluorescent tubular lighting that flickered every now and then like a cheap horror movie.
The irritating flicker commanded everyone's attention.

Addicts.

I hated that word.

The facilitator of the program instructed everyone to sit next to other family members and friends in the group. Other people.

More strangers.

What were we doing there?

The place was for other people.

I remember feeling naked and vulnerable. I broke contact with my husband and chose a seat furthest away from the entrance and as close to the back wall as possible. I kept my gaze downward toward the torn carpet. I wanted the sheet rock behind my chair to swallow me up and make everything go away.

It didn't.

I was still there.

Reluctantly, I convinced myself to lift my head and look around the room at all the sad and lost expressions. It was then that I realized that "they" looked like me.

I looked like "them," the other people.

I felt like I was treading in deep water within a sea of strangers. I needed a familiar presence that belonged to me. I remember going over each individual face, searching for my love's face. He was my only force of strength. We were partners. I wanted to see what stranger he had chosen to sit next to. I was hoping that he could hear my silent screams, so that he could rescue me from my lonely perch. When my eyes and my heart located the father of my children, I could clearly see that he, too, was still in shock. He looked like the "others" just like I did. Oddly, I guess we belonged there, but, somehow, all I could do was hold in my burning shrieks.

Suddenly all the adolescent patients entered the room. It was unsettling, really, the number of adolescents that were enrolled in a drug and alcohol addiction program. A knot in my stomach and a lump in my throat indicated a reminder of the reality that I had been living prior to coming to know this place that was meant for others.

Or was it?

What hole had I been living in?

The obvious didn't make the situation any more believable. I was as broken as a mother could be. My daughter was as broken as any struggling adolescent could be.

How had I missed the signs?

What took me so long to see that my little girl was struggling so much that she needed to turn to substance to ease any pain?

Family Therapy Part I officially began.

More instructions were given by a facilitator. We were told to create a circle with the chairs we had just sat in. He explained to all of us that one adolescent addict would sit in a chair in the center of the circle that we visitors had just created. He then described to the group that many family members or friends of the addict would be chosen and then given a scripted line. He went on to explain that the chosen family member or friend was to approach the adolescent in the center of the circle and walk around the patient using the assigned scripted line or word that was given. The scripted line or word had to be repeated over and over, in a shouting volume while walking around and around the adolescent sitting in the middle of the circle, until instructed to stop.

Addict.

I still hated that word.

I did everything to hide my availability. I pressed myself so far down into the fold of my chair, so as not to be seen by the facilitator. With all my might, I did everything I could to suppress the silent tidal wave of tears behind my eyes. I uncontrollably began to lose every breath I had.

The facilitator explained that the exercise was supposed to educate family members and friends on what types of words and sentences an addict listens to and hears in their heads every minute of every day. Sentences issued to the family cast members were horrible. The lines that were instructed to be shouted out were "You're a loser!" "You'll never amount to anything!" "You're no good!" "You're embarrassing!" and "I wish you were dead."

The facilitator unveiled my hiding spot and pointed at me. There was no wall to make me invisible, no chair that was going to save me. I was singled out and asked to step forward and wait for my scripted line.

"You're no good."

My job was to shout those crippling words over and over and over and over toward the adolescent addict who would be sitting, alone, center stage.

I was shaking.

The facilitator again explained that we who were selected to participate in this round had to continue using the scripted word or sentence while circling around the addict until we were instructed to stop.

I clearly understood the rules the first time he had said it.

It was time to join in this most hurtful group activity.

The facilitator shouted, "GO!"

As the family members and friends circled the adolescent, repeating their assigned insults as directed, I felt as though I was going to vomit.

I could not speak. The words assigned to me would not come out. I was gasping for air and getting dizzy. All I could do was sob and sob and sob. I just followed in line around and around and around the adolescent patient in the center of the circle. My assigned words never left my mouth.

I didn't understand any of this.

I was numb.

I felt as though I had failed as a mother.

One more exercise would complete Part I of the family group therapy on that tumultuous day. The task involved another young addict taking the spotlight seat. This time, all the other adolescent peers were to surround the child in the center of the circle while blaring affirmations of hope, love, and acceptance.

The facilitator shouted, "GO!"

In a celebratory instant, with a thunderous roar, every adolescent patient in the treatment center was filling the room with nothing but love and validation that was directed completely at the chosen patient in the center of the circle.

"I LOVE YOU!"
"YOU ARE WORTH IT!"
"YOU CAN DO THIS!"
"YOU ARE WORTHY!"

My child was not alone.

Neither were we.

Yet there we were. We were the others.

Much later and in much of the reading I continually engrossed myself in, I found a story written by a spiritual author on love and forgiveness. I learned that the experience in the family therapy group that I just described from that day was nothing short of the same ritual practiced by the South African Babemba tribe. When a member of the tribe is found to have behaved unworthy or with mistrust, every other member of the tribe stops what they are doing to meet the guilty one in the village center. Each member of the tribe approaches the single member in the center, one by one, reminding the guilty individual of all the good deeds that he or she has accomplished in that lifetime. The accused is reminded of the level of love each tribe member holds deeply for him or her over and over again. The forgiving ritual can last for days before the finale celebration of reuniting the once guilty tribe member back to the rest of the tribe, making the entire group whole again.

Profound.

Part I of Family Therapy Day finally came to an end.

Everyone was told that each family would be joined with their own child's therapist. That therapist would escort us to a more private room to create a family tree. The group facilitators dismissed everyone to grab a drink or a snack and return to the group room.

I remember wanting to just go to bed and wake up somewhere else where we were one happy family.

I couldn't remember that far back.

I hungered for sleep.

We had just participated in an experience of such raw emotion. It left me feeling as though I was suspended in midair in that same musty, discolored room.

I remember my eyelids feeling like they had been stapled wide open, regardless of my fatigue. It was as if crazy glue was squirt between my lash and forehead. Looking back, I realized that maybe that feeling was a sign meant to intercept any further chance of becoming blind to the new reality I had just witnessed.

Eyes wide open.

Surreal.

I was petrified for the next exercise. I knew the history that I was being instructed to reveal in the presence of a perfect stranger.

"What happens in this house, stays in this house."

What happened next broke every house rule that I had ever been trained to obey as a child.

Think about it. You already know.

Chapter 9

Family Therapy Day, Part II

My husband and I were directed to a classroom, as I recall. The room had two dry boards with markers on the ledge, apparently for use. The therapist stood on the opposite side of the room. We were instructed to pick up a marker and face the board in front of us. With marker in hand, we were instructed to remember as far back as we could the elders in each of our own families. We were told to place the names of the grandparents or great-grandparents, starting at the top of what resembled a tree that was already designed on the board.

We both faced the dry board in front of our own "tree." Beginning at the top, we both began to scribble out the ancestor names we were familiar with. We continued downward toward the bottom of the family tree.

The therapist instructed us to identify, with a mark or written word, who the family member would be that might have had experience with trauma, alcohol, or any other substance as we grew up.

I had sunk into an imaginary cylinder where I thought I could hide the stories that I had heard throughout the years. I was mortified that the past of family members was now going to be witnessed by a stranger in plain sight. My mother would never have approved of such a public sharing of private information. Who would have guessed that the stories that I had learned about through silent whispers at family gatherings like picnics, weddings, or funerals, would have anything to do with my life on that fateful day of reckoning?

I had so many wonderful memories of the grandparents that I knew as a child, but something about that brittle marker tree glaring back at me from the dry board would prove to have a lot more information than I had ever thought possible.

Yet there we were.

This much I knew of my family heritage:

My maternal grandfather was born in 1911.

When I was young, he always had a sweet identifiable scent about him. That's how I knew it was him. I loved him.

My mother always had a level of distaste for him. She was stern with him. She had rules for him.

There was a sense of confusion for me, as a child back then. I didn't know why. I didn't understand. There were stories that little ears should never hear about their elders. How does someone explain the feeling of "backwards"?

Everything felt "backwards."

As I got older, that all-too-familiar and all-too-often scent of my grandfather would come to be known as being the sweet and sour scent of stale beer.

At some point, I would come to learn that my grandfather was physically abusive to my grandmother. Terribly so, is my understanding. My maternal grandmother had passed away from brain and breast cancer when my mom was just a young mother of one child, my brother.

The disease of cancer chose my grandmother.

I never got to know her.

The horrible stories would slowly come to light later during family gatherings, funerals, weddings and the like. Amidst the reminiscent sad stories exchanged, I would learn that my mother had endured some of the brunt aftermath of all the drinking stops that my grandfather had made along the route taken that got him home from work.
I would learn that he passed from falling off a bar stool.

Inheritance.

INHERITANCE

~~~~~~~~~~~~~~~

My paternal grandfather was born in 1900.

While I was growing up in the 1960s, he was old. My grandfather had a history of strokes. He was met by a serious stroke that left him paralyzed on one side, leaving him unable to care for himself. That would not be his last.

I remember that my heart was broken.

My dad would often visit his old homestead to check in on my grandfather, as much as the old man would allow. He would demand that my father leave his home immediately, while shouting obscenities from his front door.

I remember such events as my five-year-old self sitting in my dad's Buick station wagon. I'd be waiting for him to descend from the grand porch of his old home, also spewing hurtful words in return.

Backwards.

After many years of tending to his father, my dad would have to relocate my grandfather from the decrepit family dwelling, to live with a caregiver in the next town over. It had been getting more and more difficult for the old man to live independently since the debilitating stroke that had chosen him.

Still, my dad would have his father share holiday dinners with us in our home, transporting him back and forth from the caregiver's home.
~~~~~~~~~~~~~~~

At some point, the caregiver could no longer offer the level of care my grandfather needed. Not to mention, although I am mentioning it, from the interaction characteristics and exchanges I had witnessed eye-high from that Buick station wagon back seat window, I'm pretty sure that my grandfather could have been very mean. He reluctantly resided in a home that had no familiarity to him and no family present. My dad would have to move his father again, only this time he was to live out his last days at a nursing home, due to needing twenty-four hour care.

My dad would visit his father at the nursing home, bringing him cartons of Camel cigarettes that my grandfather demanded of him every week. I would tag along.

I loved Grandpa.

Every patient in his small community there spoke of him as though he was just a wonderful man. He always took care of the ladies by pushing their wheelchairs with his right hand as he dragged his entire paralyzed left side down the hospital sterile institutional hallways, dragging his heavy left foot from behind. The old women would say to me that he was the cat's meow. Everyone loved him.

I loved him.

I began to realize that my father had always had a level of distaste for his father, just as my mother had had for her father. My dad was stern with his father. He had rules for him, just like my mother had had rules for her father. I remember that I had had a sense of confusion.

Back then, I didn't know why. I didn't understand.

Then there were stories that little ears should never hear about their elders. I don't know how to explain it, but everything felt "backwards."

Again.

I would later learn that Grandpa, as I affectionately called him, was a physically abusive man to my grandmother, terribly so. She had passed away before I was born, so I never knew that grandmother, either.

My aunt, my father's sister, would subtly tell horrible stories of her life growing up as the youngest and the only daughter. Stories like how my father would often have to jump in between his parents to protect my grandmother from my grandfather. There was a startling statement that my aunt would use when speaking of her past, "My father was not a very nice man to your dad." My aunt would rarely go any deeper into her nightmare like memories. However, when she did, I could see the trauma of her early years rushing back. It was as though she anticipated her father, my grandfather, returning home any minute from the watering hole where he spent much of his time after work. He was a factory worker.

Conflict and chaos resulted from my grandfather's frequent drinking. Explosive behavior continued for years and years. I could tell that the aftermath of such a traumatic past had forged an anger inside my father that he could never resolve. I never wanted to hear the details.

Inheritance.

INHERITANCE

~~~~~~~~~~~~~~~~

My father was born in 1933.

My father was high ranking in the local fire department and an upstanding gentleman in our community. In addition to being a fireman, he also held down a second job. He worked hard.

He was a great dad. He wouldn't raise a hand to us even if we had deserved it. Growing up was like *Leave it to Beaver* every single day. My father loved his family so much. That's how it was for us. We were so fortunate to be able to have annual vacations spent at a resort forty minutes away from our home. We went out to dinner every Sunday to a variety of different restaurants. We had Halloweens and family holidays.

My brother was the oldest, always seen in a suit. My sister, the middle child, was always in the best dresses that Sears Department Store could offer. I was the youngest of three, also touting the greatest of small child fashions. My mother always looked stunning, always chin up, with the best coiffed hairstyle, while my father was the most handsome man.

My mom was angry sometimes. I didn't know why. I didn't understand. For me, there was always a sense of confusion. There were stories that little ears should never hear about their parents.

Whispers. Silence.

I don't know how to explain it, but sometimes everything felt "backwards."
~~~~~~~~~~~~~~~~

Backwards. Again.

My dad had a regular practice of "going to the store."

Daily.

There was a tense vibe in my home that I could detect sometimes. I couldn't identify it, but something about it felt all too familiar. There was arguing, more whispers, stern speeches, threats, ultimatums, storming out, blow ups, taking sides, blaming this, and blaming that.
It became somewhat of a fabric of our woven family tapestry.

The day I got married, my father had gone "to the store" in the early afternoon. My sister and my mother were preparing for the arrival of the wedding party participants for the ceremonial pictures on the front lawn of our very small ranch-style home. I was getting my bridal hair done at a local hair salon.

My sister later told me that our dad had come home from "the store" and was completely out of control that day. She confessed that she had never witnessed such behavior before. She described feeling angry and embarrassed. The scene she painted had cried out an experience that was downright hurtful. She had said to me that our father had returned home from "the store" drunk.

I never really received all the dirty details of the events that occurred that sacred day. After all, my memory only served up the wedding entourage arriving to the tiny family bungalow, to pose for the coveted pictures that would depict a happy family living in bliss.

My sister always took the role of protecting me. I was her baby sister. It was much later that she taught me what "going to the store" really meant after all those years growing up.

"There will be no discussing anything that happens in this house!"

We were an upstanding family.

Upstanding, if no one ever discussed what really happened behind closed doors, of course.

Inheritance.

~~~~~~~~~~~~~~~~

My brother was born in 1955.

My brother was your typical comedic young boy. He was always getting into mischief, causing fun trouble until the fun trouble wasn't fun anymore. As a teenager, he was always getting grounded for smoking, sneaking, and lying about stupid things. As he grew into adolescence, he was always storming in and storming out. There was a great degree of screaming with my parents, slamming doors, slamming books. My sister and I were always witness to conflict, chaos, tears, hiding, watching, listening, whispering, and shouting.

I remember my sister and me constantly getting asked by a variety of high school teachers throughout the years, "Is HE your brother?"
~~~~~~~~~~~~~~~~

I always denied having a brother by the time I got to the higher grades, but my sister was not as lucky. She and my brother were one year apart from each other. My brother was the oldest. My sister was next, and I was four years younger, following behind them both. I had the greater opportunity to duck the accusation of heritage, and I did, most times.

Both my parents worked for the city. My dad sweated along at his second job.

"There will be no discussing anything that happens in this house!"

We were an upstanding family.

Upstanding, if no one ever discussed what really happened behind closed doors, of course.

I'm sure you know where I'm going by now.

My brother was nineteen years old when he married his sixteen-year old girlfriend. He was awarded custody of his two very young boys, following the brief marriage. My mother made sure of that outcome. My mother was a great force in my nephews' lives. She always saw that they had everything they needed, and as always, my sister helped. I think I was just the young sister and aunt who made sure the boys were laughing.

As my brother entered adulthood as a single father, there were more secrets. There were more arguments. There were more threats.

My mom was angry all the time. I probably knew why. I was beginning to understand. The sense of confusion for me when I was a child was beginning to show me a pattern as an adult.

We would learn that my brother would be away from his home at night. My nephews were living in a level of disarray and confusion. There were stories that no family ears should have to hear, much less believe.

Then my brother went away.

There it was again. Backwards.

~~~~~~~~~~~~~~~

I knew that my dad had a story about swimming with his cousin in a lake or a pond. Each of the boys might have been thirteen years old. My dad had to swim towards shore because the boys had become frightened by something in the water. His cousin never made it. My dad's cousin drowned in the lake that day. My father was blamed for not rescuing his cousin. I can only imagine what had happened behind closed doors that fateful day when my dad and his father returned home. That had to be traumatic.

~~~~~~~~~~~~~~~

My brother was living with me in 2014. He was dying from cancer. Out of the blue, as we sat quietly together, he stared into space and said, "She always blamed me." I remember responding with surprise, "Who blamed you and for what?" Still staring into space with a foggy glare, he told me a story.

He and his friend from the neighborhood were thirteen years old. They were always making fun of their sisters, ringing doorbells the night before Halloween, and doing what most kids were doing in the '60s, like playing the game of Kid Army. Once, the boys were playing that game of Army just around the corner from his friend's house. My brother told me that he had a tube of wax and, in all good, clean fun, he etched into the sidewalk the words "YOU DIE."

Shortly after that adolescent stunt, a fire broke out in the middle of the night at his friend's house. His friend was trapped and never made it out of his upstairs bedroom, consequently keeping him from leaving the engulfed home.

The boys were just thirteen years old.

A little piece of my brother died that year. He confessed to me, while telling that story, that he harbored the deep belief down in his heart that his friend's mom had blamed him for those waxed letters engraved on the sidewalk, not so many days before the unfortunate fire.
A fire my father helped put out while on duty.

That had to be traumatic, two-fold.

~~~~~~~~~~~~~~~~

My daughter was thirteen years old. So was the young man that fancied her, and she did him. They were freshmen in high school. As the story goes, the young man was at a community fair. He was walking along the very busy street to get to the car that had taken him and his friends to the fair. A car hit him, head on, as he walked. He died instantly.
~~~~~~~~~~~~~~~~

My daughter was never the same. That had to be traumatic.

If this was inheritance, my kid never had a chance.

~~~~~~~~~~~~~~~

As Family Therapy Day came to an end, the three of us found each other somewhere within the crowds of all the other families.

I was exhausted.

As I walked towards my daughter, I took a deep breath, hoping to find the oxygen that I was sure had left the room. I kept blinking my eyes to disguise my sorrow as I snuggled her soft brown head of hair under my chin. I kissed her head and told her how much I loved her. Her dad held us both so tightly.

She said, "Thanks for coming."
~~~~~~~~~~~~~~~

INHERITANCE

Chapter 10

Break. The. Chain.

No one ever said that change is easy. As a matter of fact, none of it was or is, for anyone going down the unchosen path of the Disease of Addiction. To be honest, when the most realizations of truth confront you and you face them head on, they are much uglier and harder than one would expect.

I learned that the person struggling from the Disease of Addiction has got to let go of the "people, places, and things" that have influenced the costly exchange of oneself for the lie for the high. It's a requirement to be able to begin to reprogram the brain that has been taken hostage. Life must be relearned more constructively for everyone involved. Relationships that the Disease of Addiction has stolen from everyone, must begin to rebuild from the very bottom upward to understand the healing process to be able to begin the road to recovery.

Costly exchange.

 Who wouldn't give that kind of support that is so desperately needed for those who are affected by cancer, heart disease, kidney disease, or any disease, for that matter?

Life as anyone knows it is morphed by the demand for secrecy for those living through the Disease of Addiction. The societal stigma is too much to bear. Is it possible to understand that the private information held so close to the vest by those struggling is already feeling ashamed, embarrassed, and perceived as the sole failure of the family that loves each other so much? Aren't we all a little bit embarrassed, maybe feeling as though we have failed anyone and everyone around us? When everyone in the encompassing sphere of society and community probably knows, but we deny anyway.

"What happens in this house, stays in this house!"

Suddenly, everyone must admit, agree, or at least come to terms with the fact that everyone takes a role, and not just the active user who struggles. During those reawakening times at family therapy from treatment centers, Al Anon meetings, family support groups, therapists, church, and good friends that I could lean on, I know I always said out loud, "Great, she got to get numb. I got to get crazy."

But it was crazy, and not just for me.

Talk about the Disease of Addiction OUT LOUD.

Yes. It's possible.

In my case, I was never a good enabler. I was an enforcer. I have never liked playing a hostage to anyone or anything. Not taking the enabler role did not make me any better or worse as the horrific battles, exchanges, and four-letter words were played out just about every night. We had a business in a community in which we were very much involved. As the years rolled by, I would swear that money was disappearing from our cash register on the days that my youngest daughter had come in to work at the desk. She began to ignore strict curfews. She was failing to show up to classes, and there were teachers that allowed her to leave class because they thought that she was "cool."

I became embarrassed by the secret behavior.

Then I was angry.

You might say that I became the enemy of the people.

I had called for a hearing with the teachers' union, along with the high school principal, to demand strict boundaries for my daughter. I felt that there was a teacher trying to play "parent." Something was going on so incredibly wrong, and somehow it was going unnoticed.

Or was it?

Yes, I even went as far as calling the parents of my daughter's friends.

Like the time she had been dropped off home by a friend of hers one night. She was intoxicated. Her friend and she had been at a restaurant a few miles away, and they were getting served straight vodka at the age of sixteen. I was livid. I picked up the phone and called her friend's parents. I informed the mom that my daughter was throwing up in her bathroom from alcohol and had been dropped off by her daughter. I was warning her that her daughter may also be driving home intoxicated.

The mom hung up on me.

Yes, that restaurant heard from me, too. Serving alcohol to underage children is illegal in some states. The person who is responsible for that act should get fired. And yes, again, I made sure the waitress who served the underaged patrons lost her job.

As our lives became more and more out of control, you could probably say I became a bit of a lion. The decisions I made that brought attention closer and closer to the truth, gained me no friends, but one thing that can clearly be said is that I was no enabler. I might have been a lion protecting her cub, but I was no hostage to the Disease of Addiction. And I would do it all over again.

Deep down, we all know the truth.

What was the role assigned to you?

The Disease of Addiction CHOOSES.

SOMEONE.
ANYONE.
THEN EVERYONE.

Chapter 11

My Brother Said, "Write Letters."

As much as many of the signs of a struggle with addiction are the same and relatable to those who endure the heredity, the trauma, the confusion, the darkness, the gray area I refer to, the one thing that everyone remembers with picture-perfect clarity is the day recovery began. I cannot say what day, what week, what month, nor what year that the poisonous invasion slowly made its way to us and planted itself right into our address. I can say for certain that on March 2, 2005, the healing began for our family.

The transformation from out of the darkness and back to any flicker of light required all hands on deck. Returning to the light was like unpeeling an onion, one layer at a time and with those onion skins comes the inevitable tears. A slow process at best, with a multitude of challenges to encounter along the way. That was just the tip of the iceberg. We all became desperate to find our own truth while dredging through a tsunami of therapeutic exertion, to then find our own reflection within the parts of the intricate puzzle.

One day at a time.
One letter at a time.
We did just that.

~~~~~~~~~~~~~~~

March 10, 2005

Sweetheart,

I am typing because you know what my penmanship looks like...well, it looks like yours. So, I am typing.

I can only relate to your situation in the same terms as when I quit smoking cigarettes. There were lots of habits and rituals and chemical addictions to have to put behind me. There are lots of habits and rituals and chemical addictions that you have to put behind you. It took me years to decide to quit. I spent years trying, but one day I finally decided. (A decision made in part to prodding by you and your sister, who were learning all about the dangers of cigarettes at your elementary school, coming home daily and ragging on me. I don't know if I ever told you but thanks for the motivation to make me quit.)

One thing I learned at that time was the difference between "deciding" to quit and "trying" to quit. Every time I tried, I failed. When I finally decided, I succeeded. Somebody described it to me by using the simple scenario of ordering a glass of water in a restaurant.
~~~~~~~~~~~~~~~

No customer says to the wait staff, "I'd like to try to have a glass of water." No customer says to the wait staff, "Try to get me a glass of water." The wait staff never says, "I'll try to get you a glass of water."

The customer decides, "I want a glass of water!"
The wait staff says, "I will get you a glass of water!"

With recovery, you are both the customer AND the wait staff. In the simple scenario above, you can substitute the words "glass of water" with the words of recovery.

You are strong and smart. You have a solid sense of right and wrong. You have lots of tools in your toolbox already. You are collecting more tools now. If I can help you use them better, I'm there for you.

I love you and I know you can do it.

Love, Dad.

~~~~~~~~~~~~~~~

March 15, 2005

Hey Baby,

I am a mother desperate to understand your thoughts, and you are refusing to speak with me. I spoke with your counselor on the phone. She had used the words to me, "Ma'am, your daughter doesn't want to speak with you." That's all I could hear in my head. Repeatedly, like a bad dream. This is all a bad dream. I am in no other position than to begin to understand how much of a control freak I am. I feel defeated, powerless.
~~~~~~~~~~~~~~~

Someone else has my daughter and I cannot help but feel broken. I am sure this is also, by therapeutic design, my therapy. This is a family disease, and this must be where I am accountable, where I have contributed. This feels "opposite."

I don't know if you knew that I had not been speaking with your uncle. He and I had had a falling out, as we sometimes did, over something that must have been so ridiculous; I couldn't even remember what it was about. I thought, for the very first time, I needed him. I needed to know from his recovery state of mind why you refused to speak to me. I dialed his phone number. As the phone rang, I could hear myself breathing in the receiver.

"Help me," I said when he picked up the phone. I begged him to describe to me what you were thinking and what you were doing while at this 28-day treatment center. I cried so hard; I couldn't catch my breath. He understood completely.

He has been in recovery for 18 years. You knew he was an alcoholic and cocaine addict. Long before 18 years ago, lots of feelings had been hurt, relationships lost. Communication had ceased. The day you were born, 17 years ago, he called me at the hospital for the first time in a year and asked me if he could come visit his new niece. He was sober then, too. I was thrilled to hear from him and welcomed him to visit. My brother was back in my life, in our lives.

Today, I needed to understand what you and he feel like and what my role in helping you should be. His suggestion was simple. He encouraged me to continue to write letters to you. He told me to leave you alone and that one day you would read them. He said that you were going to be alright and that this moment in time would pass. He told me to save each letter and that I would know when the time was right to share them with you.

I love you. I miss you terribly. Stay strong.

Mom.

<p style="text-align:center">~~~~~~~~~~~~~~~</p>

Friday March 18, 2005

Dear Love,

Today was a long day, as I am sure it was for you. Dad and I couldn't wait to see you and meet with your counselor for our 9:00 am appointment. After a complete traffic hold up on Route 84, Dad and I are hours late for the appointment. We finally arrived and learned that your counselors can no longer offer you treatment. The report is that you have chosen to stop eating, and as much as you try to convince your favorite therapist that you promise to eat, you are unable. Anorexia. The clinical team describes to us that by giving up one addiction, it is not unusual that another addiction is practiced replacing the original. The team explains that their facility is only equipped for substance abuse rehabilitation and not eating disorders.

I'm dying.

You came into the office, where dad and I were eagerly waiting to see you, although I felt as though you completely dismissed us as being in the room. Your clinicians deliver the news that you will soon be discharged, along with their recommendation to an Eating Disorder Unit another 2 hours away. We are instructed to drive back to our home and wait for the call that informs us that there is an "available bed," another term I have grown to hate. You leave the room angry.

I am empty.

We learned that you smoke cigarettes. As I state my complete distaste for the allowance of adolescents smoking cigarettes, it is brought to my attention that I should weigh the picture, cigarettes vs. cocaine. I cannot believe that suddenly I am grateful for cigarettes.

Dad and I got back into the car and drove back home. I am so afraid.

It was about 4:00 or 5 pm when we arrived home. The phone was ringing as we approached the back door. I ran to the ring. It was the treatment center reporting that a "bed had become available."

I hate that term.

We were instructed to come back to the facility to transport you to the other clinic immediately. Without hesitation, we did.

We arrive for your discharge and find you very angry. I feel like I am watching a television show. It is all so surreal. I want to understand. I cannot speak.

I wish I understood.

Dad secured the doors of the car; child-locked for fear that you were going to jump out and injure yourself as you thrashed around in the back seat. We drove 2 hours for your admission to a unit specializing in eating disorders.

I am numb. I cannot feel my face.

How did we get here?

We arrived. Your belongings are searched, and I feel so uncomfortable. You denounce your belief in God. You completely dismissed me as I tried to comfort you. You're my baby and I want to take care of things. I find an emotion that gives me what strength I have left to walk away from your hurtful actions.

I am broken.

Soon you faced me tearfully. You apologized, and I suddenly realized that I need to stay strong as your mother, as well. It comforts me to know that you are still in there. You showed yourself just then.

I know you're in there.

You have completed the admissions process well after midnight and begin your next phase of rehabilitation from anorexia. Dad and I arrive home at 3:00 am. I was awake the entire drive home, I bet you don't believe that. Well, I was.

I love you. We love you. Please come back whole.
Mom

~~~~~~~~~~~~~~~

Saturday March 19, 2005

Dear Sweetheart,

Somehow, I got up and went to work this morning. I need to stay connected to routine. That's how I think I am coping. I hope you had a good night, and I continue to imagine how you are doing. What are you doing? I feel completely helpless. Why are you so angry with me? You stormed away from me last night as we sat waiting in the admissions
~~~~~~~~~~~~~~~

department. Do you honestly expect me to let you starve yourself? I'm your mother. I love you. I am not equipped to even know how to help you with whatever it is that has taken over the beautiful young girl that played softball, won coloring contests, and made everyone so happy just for stepping into the room. I can't help you, and I hate myself for not being able to.

I came home from work at about 3:15 today to find Dad with the phone in his hand at the garage door. He motioned to me that you were on the phone and that I should not attempt to speak to you. Picture that.

Dad passed the phone to me. It was so great to hear your voice. You needed me as you asked me to come pick you up. You told me that you were sorry for everything. You said that you didn't belong there.

I'm sorry. The next thing I did was one of the hardest things a parent can do. I told you that I could not help you. I hated myself for that. I told you that you were in a safe place and that we would visit every day if it was allowed. I told you that I had already spoken to your sister who was looking forward to seeing you. I said that I knew how strong you truly were, and I knew that you could beat this demon but that you needed to be in the hands of professionals that would know how to help you get better.

You hated me.

I hated myself.

I listened to you cursing me with four-letter words and I told you I loved you.

Because I do.

I hung up.

I promise we will see you tomorrow. I promise. I never break my promises.

I love you.
Mom.

~~~~~~~~~~~~~~~~

Sunday March 20, 2005—Palm Sunday

Dear Sweetheart,

Your sister is as confused as we are. My heart breaks for both of you.

College is an easy escape for her. I try to figure out if that's good or bad. She thinks she is free of the questions that taunt her heart, her mind. When she lives only a short reprieve. Deep down inside, she knows that. That's why she stays there. I think she misses what was, or what she thought "was." The fact is that suddenly it became real that our lives were being controlled by something that none of us had any say in. Where did life, as we knew it, cease and life with drug addiction begin? Funny, how a substance can control an entire family; so powerful, so unfair.

We all feel betrayed, and it's apparent that your sister needs something to blame.

She wanted to come to hospital with us to visit. We walked into the grand entrance to the hospital and went up to the unit for eating disorder, a lockdown unit. So scary. So medicinal.
~~~~~~~~~~~~~~~~

I brought an Easter Basket for you. The nurse on the unit asked me why I felt the need to reward you for your behavior. The question took me by surprise. I explained that Easter was coming. I wanted to share the holiday with you as we are living a day at a time not knowing when you will be home with us. The nurse slightly recoiled and allowed me to give it to you. I am beginning to understand that we are all receiving a behavioral education as we emerge from the cloud that has hovered over us for so long.

We met you and saw that you were carrying all your belongings, which wasn't much. Earlier today, you had described that once woken up in the morning, the bedroom doors were locked until evening, leaving you needing a bag to carry any activities for the day, your books, pads, schoolwork. Other patients seemed to walk, as if in a trance, through the only 2 hallways that screamed a darkness we are all sharing. I brought you a bookbag, and you were grateful.

Most times I cannot breathe.

How did we get here?

Dad and I witnessed our 2 favorite sisters talking and laughing. It appears the four of us have accepted what has been dealt to us. For a moment, it felt like there was light.

Visiting hours were over. I don't think any of us knew what to do but to go along with the rules.

Say goodbye.

I hugged you and whispered in your ear, "You can do this. Be strong. I love you."

As the 3 of us exited the eating disorder unit, the door slammed behind us— locked. We stood there for a moment, staring at the door with its speaker and a button for access to communication to the other side. Speechless, we turned to proceed to the outdoors, although, somehow, we were in as much a prison as it must have felt for you. Neither one of us shared a word as we walked to the car.

How did we get here?

Your sister sobbed.

Stay strong, my lovely. I love you.

Mom.

INHERITANCE

Chapter 12

No Coincidences

Anyone who might know me would know that I do not believe in coincidences. I never have. I was brought up to be Catholic, as my children were. I walked up a hill for one mile each way, every Tuesday, to participate in catechism classes. Catechism is the introduction of the Sacraments taught to children and adults in the Christian religion.
Public school kids were offered this walk-up-the-hill opportunity.

Frankly, I only remember walking that far up that hill to color in coloring books, wear a white dress to make my Holy Communion at age eight, and, at age twelve, wear a red dress to make my Holy Confirmation. I learned some prayers that I still recite to this day, but never really learned what was inside the Bible, to which I was supposed to be so dedicated. I was the only family member in my immediate family that walked to church every Sunday and returned home with the weekly honey dip donuts from the local market.

My daughters, on the other hand, went to a parochial school, as their father had. He and I both agreed that getting to know what the Bible was all about would probably be of value and that our children could benefit from. Why that experience was the furthest from the truth will have to be another book, another time.

In full disclosure, in 2005, with the transformation we were all involved in, I knew I needed to return to the proverbial sanction of my Lord, just as I had dedicated my Sunday mornings to as a child.

I needed to believe in something, so I began my solo Sunday jaunts to eight a.m. Mass.

Upon arriving and taking the same seat in the same pew, in unison, I would recite the prayers I knew with the rest of the parishioners.

Each week I would grab the church bulletin on my way through the towering wooden doors. I would hold a tissue so tightly in my hand that my fingers were red and the tissue a mess. I wanted to catch every leak that my eyes seemed to produce way too often. I didn't want anyone else to become aware of my own suffering. I would become so overwhelmed when the entire congregation was directed to turn to your neighbor and "offer the sign of peace." That would be the time in the weekly service when one was expected to look another person in the eye with a gesture of kindness, love, and acceptance. How could I possibly look someone directly in the eye with warmth and support when I felt like I was suffocating and gasping for air?

I couldn't accept myself.

I would look over the bulletin's current news and parish volunteer options offered within its pages. I found my eyes drawn to brief sentences that were laid out before me at the bottom left-hand corner of the first page. It was called "A Family Perspective." The piece consisted of three or four sentences, a very short affirmation, used to remind parishioners of family strength, love, and support.

In. Plain. Sight.

The messages were profound.

I remember thinking with utter amazement, "Wait a minute. Is God speaking to me right here, right now?"

God, or maybe someone else's God, maybe a higher power or Spirit, whomever, whatever, was speaking to all of us.

Maybe the statements you are about to read are just messages.

The messages are not religious. Each message is about everything that has been robbed from those that became part of the ripple effect that is posed upon all who struggle throughout a disease. What began as the one chosen to bare the ugly monster that slays the brain every minute of every day, with nothing but constant lies of low self-worth, non-trust for anyone, no strength or love for anything but the substance, ultimately infects everyone minutely close to them.

Drink in the ultimate heartbeat of each line. Take a moment to soak up the message. Regain all that we had lost sight of while we were living in an unforgiving space that I call the gray area. Maybe we do find our way back.

~~~~~~~~~~~~~~~~

"A Family Perspective."

Family is the place to act like Peter and try to do what seems impossible—to walk on water. Our family is there to catch us, to encourage us and to stretch out a hand to save us as we dare to be all we think we can be. In imitation of Jesus, a Christian family constantly says, "Fear not!"

~~~~~~~~~~~~~~~~

Today's gospel is about SEEING. Jesus "saw Mathew" and accepted him. But the "Pharisees saw Jesus" and wanted to change him. How we see others, especially in our families, is our choice. If we "see" them as a problem, we will treat them as a problem; if we see them as a gift, we will treasure them.

~~~~~~~~~~~~~~~~

Jesus tells us today that "whoever receives you receives me." Our homes must be places of hospitality, not only to strangers, but for each other. Hospitality is not only a social grace; it is a Christian act where God is present. Hospitality brings heaven to earth.

~~~~~~~~~~~~~~~~

The mother in today's gospel would not give up. She pushed through the crowd, humiliated herself, begged and argued for the sake of her child. She did not give up on Jesus, she did not give up on her ability to get His attention, and she did not give up believing in her child's recovery. Persistent parenting is the bedrock of family stability.

~~~~~~~~~~~~~~

READ THE FIRST LINE CAREFULLY.

If God brings you to it, He will bring you through it.
Happy moments, praise God.
Difficult moments, seek God.
Quiet moments, worship God.
Painful moments, trust God.
Every moment, thank God.

~~~~~~~~~~~~~~

Jesus put Peter in charge of the Church and expected him to be a leader even though he was imperfect. Every parent is imperfect, but Jesus expects us to lead our family despite our personal faults. Imperfection is not an excuse to neglect our role. It is our challenge.

~~~~~~~~~~~~~~

The successful spouse or parent has learned to "lose their life in order to find life." Giving of oneself is a decision to make my wants secondary to others in my family and is not to be confused with "giving-in" or "giving-up." Today's gospel could be paraphrased: "What profit is there if you get all you want but lose the relationships in your life?"

~~~~~~~~~~~~~~

Forgiveness is critical to a healthy life. By holding onto an injury, we are hoping for a better past which will never happen. Forgiveness recognizes that we were unjustly treated and that it will not be corrected. Forgiveness does not condone injustice. It is a decision to not let injustice control my life any longer.

~~~~~~~~~~~~~~~

Just like the workers in today's gospel, children often grumble "that's not fair." Parents respond to children according to their needs. Parents aren't expected to treat their children equally (for their needs are different) but equitably.

~~~~~~~~~~~~~~~

There is a good parenting lesson in today's gospel. As children face new challenges, parents need new parenting strategies. Many methods that previously worked don't make sense to children today. This Lent examine your parenting style so that you are not "putting new wine into old skins."

~~~~~~~~~~~~~~~

The gospel today challenges us to "testify to the truth." We are good at pointing out NEGATIVE truths such as the shortcomings of others. We tend to be silent about the POSITIVE truths, the many good actions and decisions others do each day.

~~~~~~~~~~~~~~~

It must have been difficult for Zebedee to watch his sons walk away and follow Jesus. It was the end of "Zebedee and Sons Fishing, Inc." and he surely enjoyed working each day alongside his boys. Our children are never ours. They are only on loan to us. We raise them to let them go.

~~~~~~~~~~~~~~

A parent is meant to be a "witness to the light." To be effective, light must be in front of our children, not behind them. A parent must lead, not follow to "make straight the path of the Lord" for their children.

~~~~~~~~~~~~~~

In today's Gospel, Jesus was at home when He forgave and healed the paralyzed man. In our homes, forgiveness can heal broken relationships. Families who don't forgive are doomed to paralysis. Don't accept paralysis, forgive one another.

~~~~~~~~~~~~~~

As my weekly Sunday ritual continued, I remember a woman whom I became familiar with. Like clockwork, she and I would take our righteous place in the same pew at the same service. We would look in each other's direction to offer a recognizing nod and a smile, as if, somehow, we shared a sort of kindred spirit. One Sunday, I entered the grand arched wooden doors and took my place in the space I selfishly claimed as my pew. I looked over to where I had seen the weekly stranger whom I, oddly enough, had become to look forward to greeting with a nod and a smile.

I couldn't find her.
~~~~~~~~~~~~~~

My attention was then taken to the weekly bulletin that spoke to me Sunday after Sunday with the encouraging words from "The Family Perspective." The weekly affirmations were beginning to convince me that hope, love, and faith might just be possible for the future days ahead.

Suddenly, my trance was broken when I felt a stranger abruptly take the seat beside me. The stranger was in the space that I had claimed as my own Sunday imaginary sacred bubble. I remember feeling disturbingly intruded upon.

Trespasser.

My eyes grew wide. I shot an immediate view to my left as the rest of myself faced straight ahead. Much to my shock, the stranger that had just crossed over into my world was the woman from across the way. Her look appeared to resemble something familiar to me. Was it sadness? Maybe it was fear. Whatever it was, in that split second of landing in my secluded isolation I was forced to face the newcomer to my left. The stranger looked me straight in the eye as though wanting something from me.

She did.

She whispered that she wanted to ask me a question. I so wanted to be comfortable in that moment of personal space invasion that I had claimed as my own safe space for sixty minutes a week. There was no hesitation from her to spew her blatant curiosity.

"Why have you dropped out of sight?"

She didn't look familiar to me. Or did she?

With somewhat of a mumble, as though she felt uneasy or unsettled, she went on to explain that she had been a volunteer within our community like I was, and she noticed that there was a void of my consistent involvement in various non-profit events.

The hair on the back of my neck peaked. I was embarrassed that I had apparently blocked everything in my life's existence prior to our family's intimate relationship with the Disease of Addiction, in one way or another.

I took a deep breath and decided that lying was probably not a good idea in anyone's pew, in anyone's church, in any sacred place where folks find themselves seeking refuge week after week after week from whatever demon that anyone is battling to slay that day, that week, that year, or that lifetime.

I sat up straight, turned myself entirely toward her direction. I took a deep breath.

Breathe. Breathe.

I responded with pure honesty.

I acknowledged with a nervous smile and whispered to her in return that my youngest daughter had fallen into some difficult times and that she needed my support more than ever.

My church friend's face lit up. She chuckled, as though she had been given permission to become unshackled from a relentless tether. Her eyes became watery but reflected like crystals. She took my hand into both of hers and, again, without hesitation and perfect tone, said, "That's funny, I thought it was only my daughter that went astray."

It's a ripple effect. We all take a role.

Addiction Chooses. Someone.
Anyone. Everyone.

Everything shifted right then and there.

I could feel it.

The Sunday Service took a much different turn for the better after that encounter. Each time the congregation was directed to "offer someone a sign of peace," she and I would be sitting close enough to one another. We would look each other right in the eye and would hug each other tightly.

Genuinely.

Somehow, I was freed. We were freed.

We were not alone.

Addiction Chooses. Someone.

Anyone. EVERYONE.

Chapter 13

Discharge

We had all waited a very long time for this day to come.

Discharge.

It was the day that my baby had worked so hard for. I had imagined that discharge day would be the day that she would come home "whole." The day that everything was going to go back to the way that it was, different than it had been for the last four years or so ago. What day?

Discharge.

We didn't want her to come home to the secluded abode on the second floor of our home that had made her feel so troubled. We decided to give her bedroom a "clean sweep," so that she would feel warm and loved. We began to rearrange and clean everything in our wake.

While in the act of breaching every private space she had created in the haven of her dark fortress, we discovered how incredibly sad, broken, and desperate she was truly feeling all the years prior climbing up to the very place we were all in. There were secrets that were cleverly hidden. She had managed to put on a masked front each day she opened her castle door to face a world she had felt so separated from. We removed water bottles that were filled with vodka. We cried as we found farewell letters to close friends. I suddenly recalled the morning she had come downstairs from her personal sanctuary, with bandages on both her wrists. My chest tightens today as I type, just as it did on that very morning. The experience had left me breathless and full of fear for her, for us. We did not want to lose her to anything that was full of lies, screaming at her from her head. I recalled that we rushed her to the local hospital where she was placed on a unit for seventy-two hours.

When she returned home, I wanted to understand what was happening and begged her for insight for the bandages that caused her three days in a hospital. She confessed that she had been feeling desperate and just wanted to feel different.

Discharge.

We erased anything and everything that would spark a bad memory, a dark space, or a "trigger," as it was described to us. We put a lock on any cupboard door that stored any alcohol in it. We vowed only to host dry gatherings at home. In addition, we made a request to visitors that no cash gifts in greeting cards be given or offered while our baby continued to work on her recovery program. Trigger.

In retrospect, my husband calculated that a person returning home following seven weeks of intense daily therapy had most likely endured an estimate of fifteen years of therapy sessions within seven weeks of treatment. He came to that equation based on the following information that was present in the treatment plan:

3 hours of Group Sessions per day
1 hour of one on one with a therapist
2 hours of mandatory Alcoholics Anonymous for support
6 total hours per day

49 Days would equal 294 hours of therapy.
60 minutes per hour would equal 17,640 minutes of total therapy while in treatment.
17,640 minutes divided by 45 therapy minutes per session would equal 392 total number of sessions.
392 divided by 26 weeks (based on every other week outside of treatment)

All these numbers would equal 15 years of therapy sessions and support groups in seven weeks of treatment.

Then, of course, the family treatment plan at home consisted of one hour every other week with a psychiatrist. We attended weekly family support therapy groups.

Nothing. Nothing compared to the hard work executed by a patient at a treatment center.

Discharge.

One of the most frightening days of my life was that day of discharge.

The person I had come accustomed to mistrust and not believe any word that came in my direction, was coming back home.

The truth, in plain sight, was that the person coming home the day of discharge was not the five-year-old on the train. It was not the fifth-grader who had written heartwarming letters to her mom. The person who was discharged and coming home wasn't even the troubled adolescent that left on March 2, 2005, not one inpatient treatment center, but two.

The stranger who was discharged and returning home after seven intense weeks of serious transformation, was a brand-new being. She was beautiful. She was smart. She was ours.

She was sober.

She was scared.

We were scared.

Discharge.

On April 7, 2005, a contract was drawn up and signed by the therapists for all family members to abide by upon returning home.

Contract agreements included ten answers for each of the following categories:

I am changing my lifestyle. I will not go to the following places. List given.

I am changing my friends. There are people I will not call or see. List given.

Here is a list of friends that I will spend time with. List given.

I will agree to attend five to seven AA or NA meetings a week and obtain a sponsor as soon as possible.

I will set myself and be prepared to abide by the following time limits.

When going out socially, I will inform parents of location or any changes that occur.

If I do not follow the contract, there will be consequences I may not like.

I will work in aftercare groups.

I will talk to an aftercare counselor.

I realize that increased privileges will depend on my behaviors and must be discussed with my parents, counselor, sponsor or probation.

If I relapse or I do not complete the requirements of aftercare, I agree that the recommendation of long-term residential treatment or legal trouble may follow.

A completely new version of the seventeen-year-old was coming home to re-engage into family and community life. She had kept up with schoolwork while away and was scheduled to graduate high school in just the two months that followed.

Discharge.

Our family had learned and unknowingly adapted to live the various roles assigned to us through the disease of addiction. Since 2001, we had fallen into place as addiction demands of us. We had been in a war against the enemy.

In. Plain. Sight.

We learned that addiction not only chooses the user but chooses all who surround the active addiction and all the chaos it creates. Nonusers get reeled in and experience "the crazy," while the user gets to get numb, because he or she feels crazy.

There was so much that we had to relearn within ourselves to love better, love more strongly, love ourselves again, and love each other as was intended at birth.

Birth.

Uncanny.

We had to understand that none of it would be an overnight fix, but that all of it would be worth the recovery that addiction had stolen from all of us.

Each one of us was indisputably afraid.

Addiction Chooses.
Someone. Anyone. Everyone.

Chapter 14

One. Year. Later.

March 2, 2006

Hi Honey,

It's been one year now since all our lives changed. Especially yours. I am grateful to you. I am in a healthier state of mind. I am more physically fit than I ever was. I am more accepting of others and the way that people live. Although I work on this every single day of my life, I believe I am less controlling.

I trust.

I owe most of what I am today to you.

You are my inspiration.

You are smart.
You are beautiful.
You are thoughtful and caring in every way.
You are patient.
You think.
You love.
You are a daughter, a sister, a granddaughter, a cousin, and a niece.
You are a friend.
You have become a beacon of light through all that you have chosen and
every day, you choose again.
You are comfortable with yourself.

You're home.

Love, Mom

~~~~~~~~~~~~~~~

June 28, 2006

Hi Sweetheart,

I thought we'd be past the struggle within days of your arriving home whole. I bet everyone thinks and believes that. How wrong anyone is to think that there is a "quick fix" for any of us with any of this. So Wrong.

The most obvious is in plain sight.

This is all about you.
~~~~~~~~~~~~~~~

I am just a byproduct of all the words that speak to you in your head. I am reminded of the Family Therapy Day exercise at the treatment center when those ugly words assigned to me to yell and shout repeatedly into the ear of the adolescent patients. I never knew that someone like yourself constantly wrestles to block those unfathomable, tainted, and extremely vulgar thoughts that invade the head of someone or anyone so innocent, so kind, and unfortunately so misunderstood. I cannot imagine the words that scream at you, luring you back into the darkness of deception, can convince anyone of someone or anyone's worth, when none of those ugly words are anywhere near to truth.

But that's the YOU part.

Today I am helpless. Today, over 1 year later, I think I see you still struggling.

In. Plain. Sight.

As a mom, I want to help in every way. I want to slay the monsters and demons that so unfairly prey on my little girl. I think your contentious fight to cope is no stranger to me. I witnessed this behavior not long ago. I watched you tangle yourself in a web of confusion with another unsuspecting individual who did not have your best interests at heart.

It's a mother's instinct, you know.

A mother knows when her babies aren't settled. A mother's struggle is the ability to hold back, let go, and have enough faith to sustain a hopeful tomorrow for her children.

Where had I lost you? In what way did I rob you of your independence? Will I ever understand why I think you continue to search for that motherly figure that I think you are so desperate to look for, while I am right here beside you? I think there must be a dialogue of untruths and lies that you might keep hearing in your head.

I am right here beside you.

We will get there.

Together.

Love, Mom.

~~~~~~~~~~~~~~~~

August 14, 2006

Sweetheart,

I can sense that you are struggling. I wish I could help. You always appear so together to me. I wonder if this is a cover for your true feelings. I was so glad that you joined me at the local theater to watch your sister perform in a musical production. You laughed the whole time. When I hear your laughter, I am so convinced of your serenity that I, too, feel at peace.

As you know, I have been volunteering for the outpatient center that seemed to help you in your aftercare plan. I believe in their commitment to help others as they helped our entire family. Today I had to return a costume that your sister had worn for a fundraising event that she also became involved with in the next town over, also representing the outpatient center.
~~~~~~~~~~~~~~~~

It never had occurred to me that I would have had any apprehension entering the building where your first evaluation took place that resulted in 7 weeks of residential addiction treatment for adolescents.

As I was getting off the highway exit and headed toward the evaluating center, I could sense a knot in my stomach beginning to strangle life and reality out of every step we had taken forward to rid us of the chaotic memories of the past. I was undoubtedly surprised at my body's reaction. I continued to drive closer to the address when this realization took over me as though I had no idea as to where I was headed. I turned left into the building's parking lot. I stopped abruptly to examine the parking slot that I would take. Or maybe I stopped to decide if I would take any parking slot at all.

I could not breathe.

I parked to the left because it was easy. I knew I had to get myself together. Once my composure was slightly in tandem, I was able to put on that preverbal mask. I opened my car door and realized that I was trembling and dropped my keys. I stood up, shut the car door, and, with superficial confidence, I made a strut to the front door of the building. I turned back towards my car as though that machine would pull right up to me, throw me back in, and take me home. I saw that I had left my convertible top down.

I never leave my convertible top down.

There was no turning back. I figured I would enter the building, politely place the costume on the desk with the receptionist, and make my escape. I looked up and reached for the door handle when I saw the all-too-familiar words all in capital letters spread across the front door,

"ADOLESCENT PATIENTS."

There were other words on the door, but the rest of the letters surrounding those two words were so obscurely blurred. I grabbed for the door and pulled. I stepped in.

There I was. The memory was so clear from that first day we had entered those same doors for the first time, only today my mouth was dry.

I asked the receptionist if I could leave the costume for the young woman who had issued it to your sister to represent their aftercare program. The kind receptionist reported to me that the young woman responsible for the costume wanted to retrieve it herself and directed me to have a seat, assuring me that the woman would be right there. As I took my hard plastic seat against a blue wall, I tried not to make eye contact with any of the people occupying the same chairs that we had occupied in that same sitting area just one year ago. I didn't want them to feel as though I was judging them. I knew how they felt.

I was one of them.

As I sat there waiting, I read the list of names on the wall behind the receptionist that was dedicated to individuals who were donors to the program cause. This time, this year, I knew who the names belonged to. My eyes continued to scale the small waiting space when I caught the glimpse of numerous pamphlets. All the literature was set ever so neatly in a respective holder posed for visitors to take. The information in the metal compartment included a variety of support groups, names of supportive programs for everyone involved in the family, and a plethora of phone numbers and websites to connect with for the purpose of learning how to live again with pride and without guilt or judgment.

INHERITANCE

Self-education.

I took the pamphlet that read, "To the mother and father of an Alcoholic."

The woman who came to retrieve the costume was the director of the program. We shook hands as we smiled at one another. We both expressed our gratitude. Her gratitude was for the purpose of my volunteering. My gratitude was for your life back. We were both tearing up.

Not one day goes by without my thought of you and your state of being. I know you are in a much better place than when we first took that same left hand turn into that same parking lot. I remember that day when we didn't hesitate to put our car in PARK in that very same slot.

Though today I froze, I did find my car when I walked to the parking lot, convertible top open and all. I proceeded to get in, started her up, and noticed that on the passenger seat, I had thrown down the pamphlets that I had taken. I noticed that in that pile of very valuable information, I had also pulled the 2006 AA book of meetings for you because I knew how you were always looking for current meetings.

I love you.

I am not sorry for one step that we all took, all along the way, to take you back from whatever demons were living inside you.

I guess families can relapse, too.

I would do this journey with you all over again.

Love, Mom.

~~~~~~~~~~~~~~~~

September 24, 2006. Sunday.

Hey Honey,

I guess I heard what I had been waiting for.

You had just pulled into the driveway, returning from your Sunday AA meeting, and I was outside in the front yard, beginning my spring planting. You said, "Hey Mom, I thought of you today at my meeting."

My quick thought was, "Is that good or bad?" I've learned to stay quiet and let others speak, which is not an easy lesson for me but sometimes I am able to accomplish it if I continually practice. I have grown accustomed to sitting on the edge and entering the unknown. This time it was you who was doing the talking, and I made sure I listened.

Intently.

You told me that the discussion at the meeting was pertaining to a young girl who was telling her story. The young girl's story was based on her introduction to a church by her mother. I believe the young girl had the same name as you.

You told me that your friend was ashamed of the fact that her mom appeared embarrassed to introduce her daughter, your friend, to an audience of people from her church. The introduction ceremony that your friend was explaining to you was a type of formal announcement for
~~~~~~~~~~~~~~~~

new parishioners to your friend's house of worship. You explained that this was a big moment at this church and that your friend couldn't help but feel ashamed of her own appearance, which she felt added to her mom's ill ease.

Then you told me how grateful you were that I had never made you feel ashamed of anything. You said that sometimes you don't realize how "okay" I really am and that you were just grateful for never having to feel uncomfortable.

I was speechless.

I thought, "This is it. It's the proverbial peeling of the onion; one layer at a time."

You went into the house as I continued to plant, waking up to the fact that I could feel this perpetual smile that stretched across my face from one side to another as I dug in the dirt. Here I was, planting new life into my flower bed in the front of our home, perennials, no less. The colors would forever express their richness and speak comfort to anyone who was lucky enough to drive by and breath in the sweet aroma of such beauty.

You were growing.

Our family was growing.

No Coincidences.

You then came bounding back out from the house and jumped back into the car when you remembered another part of another story from that meeting you had just attended. Apparently, the discussion at the meeting became about different religion practices. This other friend had shared with the group about being raised in the Catholic Church. She told of a memory that while preparing to make her Confirmation, which is when one is announced as an adult to the parish, her mother and she could not agree on the confirmation name that your friend was to choose. In the Catholic faith, the confirmation name is expected to be that of a saint. It was then that you felt the need to share in the meeting that your confirmation name choice was "Barbara," simply because you were a huge fan of an ever-so-famous legendary singer/actor. In that same discussion, you went on to describe how at the meeting, many began asking you how it was that your mom would or could endorse such a choice for a saint's name if we were Catholic. I don't know what your response was during your meeting, but I do know and clearly recall that you kept stressing how grateful you were to have me.

When you started the car, I asked if I could ask you a question about the topics at your meeting. I knew how vitally sensitive it is to keep anonymity in such group settings and discussions; however, you agreed. I asked if your friend had felt so ashamed to begin with, regarding her appearance, which I was guessing had to be drastically different from the population of people at her church event, wasn't that about your friends own choices? I then asked you why your friend hadn't chosen to prepare herself with a better presentation to help her confront and overcome her own fears in front of such a crowd.

Your response taught me another thing about how our home was changing. You went on to say that there were lots of honesty issues within the family of your friend. You stated that your friend's family had no idea that she even attended or was involved with anything to do with AA.

My heart filled up so. I was torn between feeling sorrow for your friend, while I was also so emotional about our own state of honesty that we had all committed to live by and work so hard at maintaining. The state of honesty has truly set us free. I believe that acceptance of all kinds can only set us free. There is light at the end of the dimmed tunnel, beginning to get brighter and brighter one day at a time.

By the way, would you like me to tell you why I supported the choice of the confirmation name of "Barbara"? I knew that you were one of the biggest fans, and if feeling spiritual meant that you chose the name of someone whom you believed to be a saint, then that was all I needed.

I love you.

Love, Mom

~~~~~~~~~~~~~~~~

Let Go. Live Life.

The Let Go Poem ~ Miracles in Progress

To let go does not mean to stop caring,
> *it means I can't do it for someone else.*
To let go is not to cut myself off,
> *it's the realization I can't control another.*
To let go is not to enable,
> *but allow learning from natural consequences.*
To let go is to admit powerlessness, which means
> *the outcome is not in my hands.*
To let go is not to try to change or blame another,
> *it's to make the most of myself.*
~~~~~~~~~~~~~~~~

To let go is not to care for,

    but to care about.

To let go is not to fix,

    but to be supportive.

To let go is not to judge,

    but to allow another to be a human being.

To let go is not to be in the middle arranging all the outcomes,

    but to allow others to affect their destinies.

To let go is not to be protective,

    it's to permit another to face reality.

To let go is not to deny,

    but to accept.

To let go is not to nag, scold or argue,

    but instead to search out my own shortcomings and correct them.

To let go is not to adjust everything to my desires,

    but to take each day as it comes and cherish myself in it.

To let go is not to criticize or regulate anybody,

    but to try to become what I dream I can be.

To let go is not to regret the past,

    but to grow and live for the future.

To let go is to fear less and love more

Chapter 15

Talk. Out. Loud.

Our small family committed to talk to each other aloud about our own experiences with addiction and dysfunction that we unknowingly took part in during those horrific years. We vowed to be nothing but honest with one another, because that's how trust is rebuilt back into the fabric of our being.

Our lives changed.

We celebrated her high school graduation. We all found comfort in our own support systems. We welcomed a new human into our lives, called a sponsor, who sat right next to me during the graduation ceremony.

Her sponsor grasped my hand and held on tight throughout the pomp and circumstance, as I did nothing but sob. This gift of a human was wise enough to know that I was having a difficult time with sadness, celebration, pride, and the overall awareness of where we were and how far we had come. I couldn't see through the stream of tears that took over my eyesight. We were all growing to understand the depths of what it takes to conquer, accept, give, understand, and love each other again.

Our youngest daughter became a public speaker, sharing her story and her meaning about strength, hope, and addiction recovery to audiences. She sustained employment working in adolescent group homes, caring for children who had been abandoned or removed from their homes through a child protective state system, the same system that made a home visit to our home back so many years ago.

My baby, although not a baby anymore, moved forward and took the glorious path to help children who were unfortunately or fortunately taken away from their families. Her strength was finding happiness and hope in a situation that no child has control over. Some of the children were granted permission to join our family for holiday dinners.

Our lives changed.

I cannot express the positive changes that have been weaved within all of us. None of which was easy, and certainly none of it was a quick fix to all that needed fixing. Sisters became best friends. Cousins became proud of each other. Grandparents could not believe the transformation we were all undergoing. The butterfly emerged from the darkness of the caterpillar's cocoon.

The day of the high school graduation party, we hosted a completely dry afternoon, as we promised in the family contract. We had great food, soft drinks, and volleyball with her friends that she committed to stay in contact with per her portion of that signed discharge contract.

My mom most undoubtedly wanted to join everyone to celebrate the high school graduation and was not going to miss it for the world; however, attending our gathering was difficult for my mom. I knew she was going to be uncomfortable at a celebration that offered no alcohol. In her hay day, everyone offered alcohol to company, everyone drank. She was embarrassed to think about the outrageous message, the silent secret that would be exposed about the family that offered no alcohol to adult guests. What would the guests think?

It was my mom.

Back in the day, she demanded the rule be followed that "all that happens in this house, stays in this house" following each explosive event with my father, and then with my brother.

We were an upstanding family, as long as no one knew what was happening behind closed doors.

Backwards.

Stigma.

Yes, well, we were an upstanding family, and I wanted our guests to recognize growth, love, honesty, and celebration of life.

At that time, my mom began to decline in what doctors had diagnosed as early-stage dementia. I was in the kitchen preparing the picnic lunch for everyone that came to the graduation celebration, when my mom stopped me. She did not give me any eye contact, but I knew she was contemplating something. She stared. She said it. My mother whispered with great intention, "I wish I had done what you did."

In my utter astonishment of such a loving statement, I wanted to hear it again. I gave her immediate eye contact with bewilderment and asked her to repeat what she had just said.

She turned around to face me with a sadness about her, full of confusion.

She did not remember saying it. That was okay.

Positive changes.

Our daughter began volunteering with a non-profit organization that her sponsor had been deeply involved with. She earned a recognition award for her hard work and dedication. She earned a Grade Point Average of 3.82 in college while living in a dorm that she secured herself by writing a letter to the dean of the university she attended. She had made a legitimate case about her need for her own space. She made the request for a private room so as not to share a dorm with roommates who would most likely be living another type of college party life. She wrote that she had chosen recovery at a very early age and wanted to sustain a sober living.

Her request was granted. We were so proud and elated about her future.

All sounds lovely.

Nothing overnight.

None of it was easy and, most times, a daily struggle.

It's a process that continues to this day.

This day.

One day at a time.

INHERITANCE

Chapter 16

Unusual Inspiration

Unusual Inspiration ~ A Cousin Perspective

English II Pre-AP

2 November 2006

For most people the word inspiration conjures up thoughts of an infallible person who can do no wrong and works like a superhero to make the world a better place. For most of my short life, I adhered to these typical stereotypes and looked up to heroes like Olympic athletes, celebrities, and incredible doctors. I never imagined one of my biggest inspirations would have to overcome tremendous obstacles and even screw up before seeing the light.

My cousin was always four years older than me, four years better than me, and four years cooler than me. My incredible older cousin, an outgoing high school senior at the time, always had the best shoes, the most fashionable clothes, and most of the time an I-am-to-coolfor-this attitude. I thought she was going to be famous, and so did she. She could sing like no other, had an uncanny ability to produce any form of art, and even modeled. She always seemed so sure of herself, so confident and collected. Apparently, she had another hidden talent; she could hide what she was doing really well.

I can remember my mom telling me the day that my cousin went into Rehab for drug and alcohol abuse. I couldn't believe it. How could the person I used to play with, the person I had so much fun with at the beach in the summer, and one of the most perfect people I knew, have done such a terrible thing? After all, I had seen *Law and Order*. The drug addicts always came across as the scum of the earth, and my cousin was nowhere near the people they portray on television. Right then and there I knew she could overcome all the enormous obstacles she had before her. She could do it just because she had always been so strong. I never imagined my cousin would exceed the word "overcome" one hundred times over. I don't even think "overcome" is an accurate word to describe what she did.

The first time I went to see my cousin was on my fourteenth birthday. We were going to visit family and we were going to attend a graduation party for her. I was so nervous. Mind racing, butterflies churning, I finally got off the airplane and saw her. Appearing so radiant and free, I could see she was a totally different person working to change her life around. Just like a teenager never missing a meal, she never missed a meeting. No exceptions! She was even thinking about her future career and college.

When I started ninth grade, she started college. Since then, she has been working hard to become a drug and alcohol counselor. She will be able to help so many people who are struggling the same way she was. She has gone above and beyond. She is an active volunteer in the addiction field and recently received an award for her volunteering. I don't think my cousin knows how much I really look up to her. She has done something many people can't even attempt to do. She has had to deal with grown-up issues before she got to that stage in her life. I am so proud of her. I never would have thought a few years ago that an inspiration could be someone who did some wrong before they contributed their good. My cousin was just a caterpillar who turned into a butterfly a little too late. These days she focuses less on becoming famous and more on making a difference. She will be famous, though. I have no doubt. Maybe not for all the superficial things celebrities today are famous for, but for the countless amazing things she will do for other people. Watching her overcome these obstacles has helped me grow as a person. It makes me think I can truly get through anything if she can single-handedly change her life around. I hope she knows that she has someone in her life who thinks she can accomplish anything. My cousin's situation constantly has me wondering whether I could be as strong as her.

Could you?

Chapter 17

Be. The. Change.

She worked hard.

Student Information

Term: Fall Term 2009

Degree: Bachelor's Degree

Level: Undergraduate

Academic Standing:

Course Work - Undergraduate

Grade	Attempt Hours	Earned Hours	GPA Hours	Quality Points
A-	3.00	3.00	3.00	11.01
A	3.00	3.00	3.00	12.00
A	3.00	3.00	3.00	12.00
A-	3.00	3.00	3.00	11.01
A	3.00	3.00	3.00	12.00

Summary for Undergraduate	Attempt Hours	Earned Hours	GPA Hours	Quality Points	GPA
Current:	12.00	12.00	12.00	47.01	3.91
Cumulative:	50.00	50.00	50.00	191.03	3.82
Transfer:	.00	63.00	.00	.00	.00

I got involved.

I jumped in with both feet. I began to volunteer more often for the outpatient program that helped guide my daughter to her recovery. I included the family business that we had owned for almost twenty years, by hosting a mother-daughter evening. The event was created for drug and alcohol prevention by opening the lines of early communication between middle school-aged girls and their moms. Moms and their daughters were to come to our business to enjoy an evening of food, self-care, and pampering, while sharing precious time with each other to encourage a positive bond of trust.

Later, I was invited to volunteer to head the entire project. I could not have been more honored and excited to become more involved with such a purposeful program. I was fortunate to have so many community partners to help support the mission and vision of early drug and alcohol prevention. I had professional friends who opened their restaurants on a closed evening so moms and their daughters could build strong relationships. I had a professional camera gentleman who volunteered to film Valentine's messages between mothers and their daughters.

I had friends in the town park department assist me in coordinating a Flash Mob in the center of the city's park on a summer solstice evening. Everything in the planning of such a dance event is completely secretive for the shock value to an unsuspecting audience who planned to sit in the park that night to listen to a summer band.

I coordinated rehearsals in my backyard with a very small group of folks who wanted to be in on the fun of the very popular Flash Mob trend that was happening around the country at that time. My older daughter and I went around introducing the idea to most of the nonprofit organizations that supported children's programs in the hopes of encouraging families to participate in one way or another.

She and I truly did not know what to expect for the turnout of such a mystery event or what it was going to amount to. Fortunately, the featured entertainment that fine evening was also in on the mob surprise for the audience that showed up with their lawn chairs.

I remember looking at my oldest just as the cue was coming from the band. I said, "It might just be me and you out there dancing in front of all these people. Are you with me?"

A true trooper, who had solidified a great relationship with her sister throughout all the shedding of all our old snake skins, "I'm ready!" She and I held hands tight enough to cause fire red pressure marks that left a pool of sweat between our palms as we stood in wait.

My great friend, the professional cameraman, filmed the event. My husband became part of the sound mechanics for the show, and by then, my baby had become a reporter for a newspaper. She was scheduled to write about the secret shenanigans. We were all in place, waiting for the proposed ball to drop with the cue from the band.

"…you never know what's going to happen at any of our shows!" shouted the lead singer, interrupting their own performance. With that, the music that my friends and I chose from the prevention department to represent adolescents and the strengths they all possess to fight against drug and alcohol abuse, began to boom, boom, boom, then blare!

My older baby and I trotted out to the center of the grassy area, curiously looking to the right and then to the left. We looked at each other in question, when at the exact same moment, and much to our surprise, we became aware of an obscure movement coming from within the onlookers from their lawn chairs.

One by One.

Over one hundred adults, little children, teenagers, parents and grandparents, staff from the outpatient center, my dearest friends, my family members, actors and actresses from the local theater groups, many different areas of the community and non-profit arenas had all come out to join the unsuspecting amateur dance team that had been planted in secret, deep within the hearts of so many people who believed in a great cause. We were amazed and speechless as to the outpouring that had occurred in that surreal moment.

Needless to add, I remember that I began to cry. Then laugh. I forgot my choreography that I had spent weeks preparing, sharing, and practicing. The chosen song had come to an end, and everyone stood up from their own patio chairs in applause. Some folks had just thrown themselves in to dance to a song they knew. We were all hugging each other. All of us.

Yes, even the strangers.

Somehow, in just a two-minute exercise, everyone got to know one another without actually knowing one another. Today, as I reminisce that very magical moment, I still get emotional and find it difficult to have any words that would describe the phenomenon that bonded complete strangers.

It was then that I was invited to turn that one full year of volunteering into a part-time profession. I began getting paid to become a program coordinator for their moms and daughter events. While still running my business, I took the opportunity.

I became a voice to help change laws within my state.

I wrote and read aloud my personal testimony to change two state bills. One was geared toward the necessary adjustments for consuming alcohol while boating. I was challenging the contradiction of a law, known as the Senate Bill 272—An Act Concerning Drunk Boating. The law originally allowed boaters, under the influence, to stay out of reach of the authorities by staying some hundreds of feet away off the shoreline until said boat driver could gain a level of sobriety.

Written testimony Before the State's General Assembly Environment Committee, March 8, 2010. Testimony to take action on:

SB 272-An Act Concerning Drunk Boating.
Dear Honorable members of the Environment Committee,

I am a resident of the state, as well as a motor boat owner, who resides for most of the summer at a local marina. Today I am asking the committee to take action on House Bill 272.

*In June of 2009, I became a boat owner. I made a responsible choice to complete the one day, 8-hour course and successfully receive the boaters' license. Simply put: Stated on page 50 of the 2009 CT Boaters Guide that is distributed and sponsored by the State of CT Department of Environmental Protection, under Boating Regulations/Boating Under the Influence it clearly states: **"No person is to operate a boat while under the influence of alcohol or drugs. The penalties for operating a vessel under the influence of alcohol or drugs in CT have increased. The laws for boating under the influence have been amended to mirror motor vehicle law."***

Please take action to the contradictory minimal limitation to the 2-hour window to test for blood alcohol levels in individuals who have chosen not only to put my family at risk but to ignore that very demand put into print. If amending laws to mirror motor vehicle law, the length of travel time in a boat compared to a car has got to be taken into consideration. Leaving my home to travel to the marina can be a 55-minute ride by car. Leaving from the property that my boat resided and sailing to the marina took us approximately 4 hours.

Breaking the law by using any substance or alcohol while operating any watercraft should be enough to prosecute anyone. Expanding the minimal 2hour limit for blood alcohol testing would ensure proper accountability. Please stay consistent. Please send one vital message. Boaters will be held accountable when they ignore boating regulations.

*I've heard it said at drug and alcohol prevention forums that "it's alcohol's job to mess up your head." If that it is true, by all behavioral choices made that result in tragedy, let it be your job, as the power you hold, to make each person accountable within the maximum amount of time for the poor and sometimes, unfortunate **choice** a boater makes to allow any substance, drugs or alcohol, to "mess up their head." Please choose to keep my family safe.*

Thank you.

The bill was signed into law on May 27, 2010, by the governor of the state.

The second law I was successful in aiding was Bill 157—An Act Revising the Definition of a Child Care Facility to Conform with the Definition of a Child.

My testimony spoke directly to the maturity, or, in its true form, immaturity, of the brain development when a child is in active use of substances. Many studies have shown that brain development progressively declines at a possible minimum of two years for each year a person is in active substance use. Therefore, if a child is screaming for help at the age of seventeen, and that person had started substance use at the age of thirteen, the possible brain maturity level of that individual may very well be that of a nine- or ten-year-old, possibly, an eleven-year-old child.

The point being is that the substance is truly conducting all the immature talking, the arguing, the stealing, and the lying. It is the addiction that has chosen that individual. The addiction has robbed that person of being able to make any rational decision that a family would expect. The addiction has robbed everyone connected to the addict of all their trust and happiness while blurring the picture of what love looks like, what love feels like, all in exchange for the coveted secret that each person holds close enough to be blinded by.

Testimony - Bill 157-An Act Revising the Definition of a Child Care Facility to <u>Conform with the Definition of a Child</u>

Good afternoon, Representatives, Senators, and Members of the Select Committee on Children. I am here as an employee whose responsibility is to connect families to treatment. I am also a parent whose adolescent revealed that she was using substances at age 17; however, today, as an adult, she has just celebrated 7 years in recovery.

I am here to testify on Bill 157—An Act Revising the Definition of a Child Care Facility to Conform with the Definition of a Child.

I'd like to share a few facts:

Troubled Teen 101 reports that the substance abuse effects to adolescents as:

- *Slower brain and body development*
- *Loss of short-term memory and ability to learn*
- *Underdeveloped motor skills*
- *Impaired emotional and sexual development*
- *Defiant behavior and conduct disorders*
- *The inability to judge risks*

Just to name a few.

Through the Mentor Foundation.org, according to Dr. Jay Giedd (2004) and colleagues at the National Institute of Mental Health in the United States, evidence is accumulating that the brain is not fully formed at puberty as earlier thought. Rather, the brain continues important maturation that is not complete until about age 25; Annals of the NY Academy of Science, 1021, 77-85.

A conversation with an RN reported that an 18-year-old that enters into adult treatment today, as she describes it, "is a little sheep in a lion's den." The 18-year-old is more apt to find difficulty handling the emotional portion of treatment, a necessary part of group therapy that allows a participant to develop new ways of relating to people. The difficulties that bring an adult to treatment, such as job loss or family abandonment, are more severe than that of an adolescent who might not have ever left home. Therefore, an 18-year-old would benefit more with like-minded peers who are learning the necessary skills to enter into adult life by taking a look at themselves realizing where they are, in order to become productive members of society.

When my daughter's secret life was exposed as a senior in high school, based on brain development studies, her thought process was most likely that of a 15-year-old. Because on paper, she would be defined as an adult in only a few months, my husband and I scrambled to beat a calendar to ensure that she receives the treatment she needed to put her back on track within her present scope of development. We were blessed with a response and a great sense of timing that ultimately saved my daughter's life. 20/20 Hindsight, of course, but I assure you, no family is prepared when the reality is presented that the elephant in your family room has been cocaine all along.

My daughter can be your neighbor, niece, cousin, sister, or granddaughter. My daughter can be your daughter. Luckily for my family, my daughter was stopped early enough in her addiction to be able to cognitively get her life back on track. It is no coincidence that she would report to you today that she remembers, almost to the moment in her third year of sobriety, when she felt that her brain began to think like normal. She was 20 and 3 years sober.

Adults play an important role by using their judgment to protect teenagers. We do what we can at home then we turn to you, the decision makers, The Select Committee on Children. Please Revise the Definition of a Child Care Facility to Conform with the Definition of a Child—Bill 157.

Developmentally, they're still babies.

Thank you.

The bill was signed into law on June 16, 2012, by the governor.

Addiction Chooses Someone.

Anyone. Everyone.

Chapter 18

That. Was. Then. This. Is. Now.

My mom passed away.

Heart Disease chose my mother.

Because of her, I am.

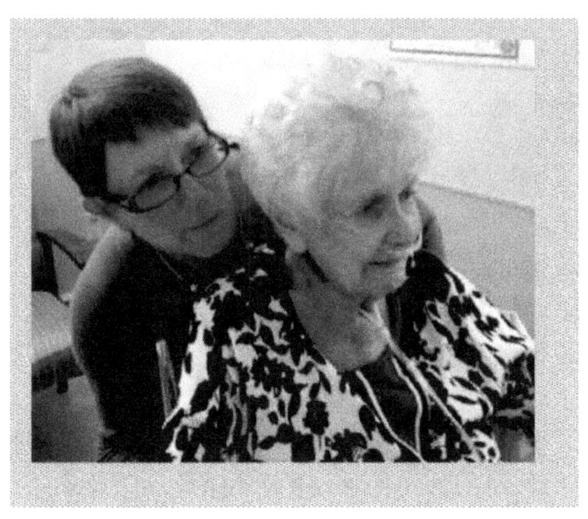

My dad and brother also passed.

Cancer chose my brother. Kidney Disease chose my dad.

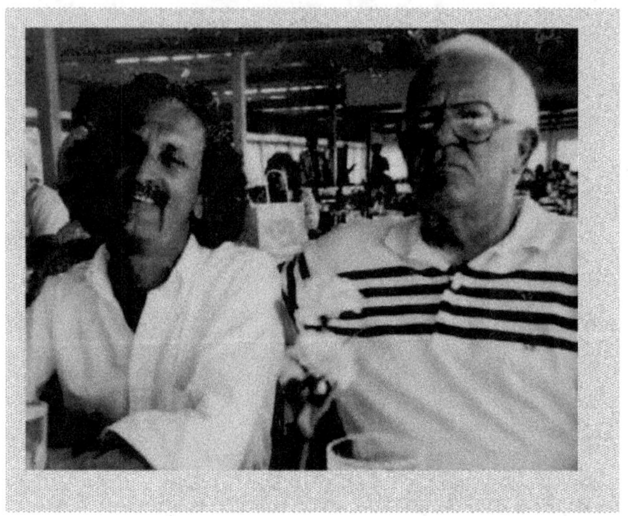

They were both over thirty years clean and sober.

Hostage to the disease of addiction.

That's what we are.

First, I was fearful and ignorant of such an ugly, invasive, most hurtful way of living. For Everyone.

 Or was it denial?

We sold the family business, and I dedicated my life to helping others in the same situation. It was a calling of sorts.

I began to work for facilities that guided families to the right resources that could offer the best path for an outcome that anyone could imagine.

Like my family.

Like your family.

For seventeen years I looked that ugly monster right in the eye. I challenged that terrifying dark serpent that chooses someone. That serpent chooses anyone.

That damn serpent chooses everyone.

But I did it.

For seventeen years, I answered calls to those that struggle. For twenty-four hours a day, seven days a week I listened to addicts; I still hate that word. They shared their plight with me. I heard them beg for help. I helped them get to the right place to start a whole new life.

Some make it. Some, unfortunately, don't.

When requested, I spoke to families at the funerals for those that succumbed to the tight hold that the disease of addiction takes on one, someone, anyone, everyone. I had never met any of the unfortunate victims, yet I spoke to them at all hours of any and every night.

The crescendo to my eulogy was for everyone who came to honor the life of the loved one who was going to be laid to their rest.

"Just pick up the phone."

 More common than anyone is willing to admit.

I learned so much through my daughter's horrific journey. I learned about her strengths. I learned about my strength. My family learned about love and strength.

In the end, which is really the beginning, I might say that I am grateful for the dark hole horror of a path that was placed before all of us. We are stronger as a family unit. We discuss topics as adults. We respect each other from all angles. We have learned our boundaries and acceptances. We all live a more joyful, productive life within our own spheres.

Love dominates.

Hostage no more to the disease of addiction?

One day at a time will tell.

Chapter 19

Once. Upon. A. Time...

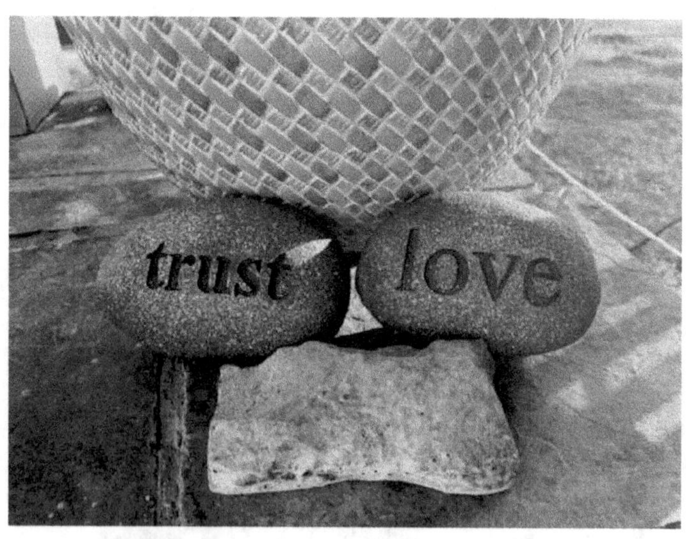

.... There is Beginning.

If this is INHERITANCE?

I am wealthy.

We all are.

Epilogue

"Then my brother went away."

I would be remiss if I did not include a beautiful letter from my brother.

I was a newlywed and didn't really understand what was going on between my parents and my brother until my mom asked me to allow my nephews to live with my new husband and I. You see, my parents and my brother agreed that he would admit to a treatment center to save himself and save his family with his young sons.

The letter refers to a note coming from me. To be fully transparent, I wish I could remember what I said in the letter to him, but I don't. I can only guess that I had disconnected with him following his discharge from that treatment center because I didn't understand back then. I'm guessing that I was hopeful that we could mend our relationship that had been disheveled during such confusing and backward times. I missed him.

One firm thought I had when I read this letter that I keep close to my heart to this day was that the "Someone" chosen by the Disease of Addiction is a human. A human struggling from the Disease of Addiction who is desperate for acceptance and connection. A human that chooses recovery over sickness, who wants to be understood and be loved in return.

Addiction Chooses Someone.

Anyone.

Everyone.

Recovery is possible.

For Everyone.

Dear Kelley

   I am so glad that you wrote that letter although I must say I was scared to open it

   I realize now how the past year was affecte everyone and for that I'll always be sorry,

   I never intentionally meant to hurt anyone most of all my own family, I never knew Erin was in the Hospitol or even sick, I heard about it weeks maybe even months later when Terry had talked to Ma and she told her, I was hurt that nobody bothered to tell me because I would have been there, I think about her all the time

   I know I am not perfect but I don't think anybody made it easy for me to feel I was apart of the family, when I went to Spofford it was to get help and coming home to find my children gone to Marijo & through my own family doing hurt, hurt more than you'll ever know, it mad me feel that none of you had any trust or confiden in me, almost like you were testing me, just waiting for me to go back to drinking so every-one could say you knew I couldn't do it,

   All I wanted was a chance instead I come home to nothing, I'm sure you all had your reasons but try to understand where I was coming from,

   I love you more than you'll ever know, I just want to be accepted for who I am, we all make mistakes but hopefully we learn from them and go on,

I WANT US ALL TO BE A FAMILY AGAIN TOO, BUT I NEED TO SEE THAT THIS IS WHAT EVERYONE WANTS AND FOR THE FIRST TIME I FEEL IT IS.

I HAVE HURT AND CRYED MANY TIMES MYSELF, FOR ALL OF US. I AM SORRY FOR EVERYTHING & TRUELY HOPE WE CAN GO ON FROM HERE.

THANKS AGAIN FOR WRITING.

Love
Paul

My dad. My brother. My baby.

Addiction. Chose. Them.

All three CHOSE Recovery.

It's possible.

www.ingramcontent.com/pod-product-compliance
Lightning Source LLC
Chambersburg PA
CBHW051745250726
48659CB00001B/253